Dr. Dan, you have changed my life and have given
of life and I could never repay you for what you ha
special talent. You have added so much joy _d
— Edward T. Allen (YFCC patient)

Dr. Dan has totally changed my life. Not only is Dr. Dan our chiropractor, but he
is our great friend, coach, mentor, and has helped us out over the past few years by
teaching us better health through awesome workshops.
— Dennis and Vicki Bruno (YFCC patients)

At the age of 41, I was able to stop taking all eighteen of my medications and am
now living a drug-free life. I am no longer a diabetic and have
lost ninety-eight pounds.
— Bryant Maulkey, (YFCC patient)

Thanks so much to Dr. Dan and his staff for their outstanding dedication and
passion for bringing the principled chiropractic lifestyle to this community.
— Carol Copeland (YFCC patient)

"As a proponent of logic, Dr. Yachter takes a systematic approach to help you help
yourself. Doctor of the Future is a progressive, take-charge book that will empower
you with knowledge and therefore the ability to take your health into your own
hands. By following the science-based advice in Doctor of the Future, you will
significantly stack the odds in your favor of leading a happy, disease-free life."
— Brendan Brazier, Professional Ironman triathlete, two-time
Canadian 50km Ultra Marathon Champion
Author of the national bestseller THRIVE and formulator of VEGA,
whole food plant based health products

"Dr. Dan knows what it takes to truly succeed in life and tells it in a dynamic and
unforgettable way. These messages and truths discussed in Dr. Dan's book, belong
in the hands of every person who wants to pursue health, happiness, and lead the
extraordinary, abundant life God has created them to live."
— Dr. Chris Zaino- MR. AMERICA, 1998, President of Abundant Life, world leader in health.

Dr. Daniel Yachter challenges the direction of the current "sick care" system, and offers a provocative alternative. If you are interested in empowering yourself to lead a radiant, vibrant, purpose-driven life, read this book.
- *Christopher Kent, D.C., J.D., Co-founder and CRO of The Chiropractic Leadership Alliance*

Dr. Yachter is the 'doctor's doctor'. His insights and immense patient care experience uniquely qualify him to assemble and present vital, common sense information that could very well save your life! The "Doctor of the Future" is something everyone should read now.
- *Patrick Gentempo, Jr., D.C.*
Co-founder and CEO of The Chiropractice Leadership Alliance

What a book! What a message! What truth! This is the single most important and timely truth for those who desire to live a long life and who desire to finish what God started.

Dr. Dan Yachter has touched my life and the lives of so many people in our church family alone. His passionate desire to see people live and feel better is one of the most encouraging signs in a changing world where commitment to helping others is no longer important. I've never met a man whose sole purpose is to live his life for others, and to see them live the greatest life. He is nothing short of extraordinary. He is my doctor and my friend, his insight and care has forever touched my life. So many wonderful things can be said about this man, but one word comes to mind when I think about him...CARING!
Now, get reading because healing is on the way!
-*Sam Hinn, Senior Leader, Pastor, The Gathering Place Worship Center*

Dr. Dan is the Doctor of the Future! He has outlined in his book the "Doctor of the Future" all the steps necessary to stay healthy and strong and free from ALL sickness and disease.

Dr. Robert O. Young, Ph.D., D.Sc., Best-Selling Author of The pH Miracle

DOCTOR

OF THE

FUTURE

DOCTOR

OF THE

FUTURE

LEARN THE SECRET STRATEGIES
THAT WILL ALLOW YOU TO RECLAIM
YOUR HEALTH AND VITALITY.

DANIEL YACHTER, B.S., D.C.

Advantage®

Published by Advantage, Charleston, South Carolina.
Member of Advantage Media Group.

ADVANTAGE is a registered trademark and the Advantage colophon is a trademark of Advantage Media Group, Inc.

Printed in the United States of America.

ISBN: 978-1-59932-156-1
LCCN: 2009914327

This publication is designed to provide accurate and authoritative information in regard to the subject matter covered. It is sold with the understanding that the publisher is not engaged in rendering legal, accounting, or other professional services. If legal advice or other expert assistance is required, the services of a competent professional person should be sought.

Most Advantage Media Group titles are available at special quantity discounts for bulk purchases for sales promotions, premiums, fundraising, and educational use. Special versions or book excerpts can also be created to fit specific needs.

For more information, please write: Special Markets, Advantage Media Group, P.O. Box 272, Charleston, SC 29402 or call 1.866.775.1696.

Visit us online at **advantagefamily**.com

Doctor of the Future is a guidebook for how

you and your family can transform American health care.

It shows you what you need to know today to take better

care of your health, and your family's tomorrow.

It also illustrates how to use the body's own

power of self-healing to produce greater

health and vitality.

PREFACE

In this book, you will learn how to get in tremendous shape in minutes a day, ways to effectively hydrate, and tips to help defeat fatigue and assist in creating extraordinary energy levels throughout the day. You will learn budget-friendly, alkaline-based meal plans, the secrets to a great night's sleep, and finally, insights on how to become non-reliant upon dangerous medications, avoid expensive medical/hospital bills, and improve your quality of life by tapping into the cutting-edge science of health and healing from the inside out. You'll discover strategies that enhance brain-body communication and maximize the function of the most important system in the human body: the nervous system.

This book is dedicated to all the patients who have put their trust and faith in me, allowing me to experience my greatest passion in life: saving and transforming lives. I thank God for using me as a catalyst to allow others to reach their full God-given healing potential and eventually their divine destiny.

TABLE OF CONTENTS

INTRODUCTION

"The first wealth is health."
–Ralph Waldo Emerson

My father is sixty-eight, healthy and drug-free. But when I was growing up, he suffered from intense migraine headaches. At times they were so bad that he'd stay in a dark, quiet room with no noise or light. He tried many drugs to help the pain, to no avail. Bottles and vials of medication spread from the bathroom to the kitchen cabinets. My house was almost like a pharmacy, and for it, his organs suffered. When the headaches were bad, my father would take a huge number of aspirin and could have ended up destroying his kidneys. As a kid, I remember my father passing painful kidney stones. Eventually, his thyroid crashed on him. He couldn't control his weight because his thyroid was not working properly, so he was always thirty to forty pounds overweight. The deterioration of his thyroid meant even more medication and expenses. His headaches continued, as they had at a very young age, and after forty years of fighting his own body he fell into despair.

This was how he lived and how my brother and I grew up; we were not familiar with alternative doctors or medical practices, but I saw how the mainstream medical institution failed him. I first encountered chiropractic when my brother, David, was in a car accident. He was a student at the University of Florida when he was T-boned by a car driven by an elderly gentleman. One morning, after a few weeks trying to recover, he tried to get out of bed only to find that he couldn't move. He was in so much pain from the accident that he felt crippled. The orthopedists and radiologists told him he was going to need spinal surgery along with pain killers for the rest of his life. At that time, my brother was twenty, in good shape, and athletic; that was the last thing he wanted to do. But in my family, we did whatever the doctors told us to do. We never questioned medical authority.

It just so happened, however, that my brother's best friend had been helped by a chiropractor. His friend explained to him what it was, and my brother, though skeptical, made a leap of faith and went to see him. In three weeks, David was restored to full health and function; he never needed the drugs and never had the surgery. The effect was nothing short of miraculous, and this sparked his interest in chiropractic.

Eventually, he was so excited he decided he wanted to become a chiropractor. He filled out an application to Life University, was accepted, and matriculated in its chiropractic program in the fall of 1990.

After a few months of school, David came home to find my father lying in his dark, quiet bedroom suffering as he had our entire lives. The familiar sight of seeing him with a pillow over his head writhing in pain and crying out to God for an answer was something he had done for forty years. My brother said, "Dad, I think what I'm learning in school is going to be able to help you." Dad had been to many specialists throughout his life, and not one had been able to help him. David had only been in school for three months, and my father was skeptical, but he had long been out of options.

David started feeling Dad's spine and he found a bone misplaced in Dad's neck—his atlas, the top bone in his neck. David asked what problem, not just treat the effects. They want to live a life of vibrant health and well-being that is drug- and surgery free. They want to experience an abundant, long life, the life that God intended for them by using their body's own optimal healing potential. This is what today's health-care consumer wants and demands.

CHAPTER ONE

THE STATE OF HEALTH TODAY

"To lose one's health renders science null, art inglorious, strength unavailing, wealth useless, and eloquence powerless." –Herophilus c. 300 B.C.

"If prescription drugs are so good, where are all the healthy drug takers?"
–Dr. Joseph Mercola (owner of the world's largest health and wellness website)

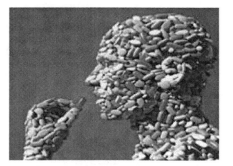

Today's health-care system has taught Americans to be reactive toward their health and not proactive. The current system does not have people asking, "How do I become healthy?" but rather, "What's wrong with me and what do I need to take to solve the problem?"

Through various marketing ploys, the capitalistic nature of pharmaceutical companies has left Americans disabled in terms of their ability to make proper decisions as to what health is and what it is not. The brainwashing comes from daily exposure to pharmaceutical commercials that have left people with a complete misrepresentation and misconception of what health is, where health comes from, and how they can actually stay healthy on a daily basis without drugs and surgery.

To further increase profit, drug companies invent disease, and subsequently offer a solution, which is nothing short of disease mongering. This is the root cause of the deadly medical lies that have been perpetrated on the American public. The lies include high cholesterol as the culprit of heart disease, the body's deficiency in Prozac as a reason for depression, and insulin as the only treatment for diabetics. Through "junk science" and "ghost writing," the public and some of the world's most respected health experts have fallen victim to these outright lies.

According to Shane Ellison, author of *Health Myths Exposed,* "Inventing disease is not a 'far-out' conspiracy theory. It is a simple matter of finding ailments that naturally occur due to poor lifestyle habits and labeling them as a disease. Once 'big-pharma' steals jurisdiction over the general public's common sense, they convince them of the necessity of their drugs."

Before coming to my office, patients typically rely on drugs and surgery. However, our bodies are designed and created the way the Creator designed them—to rely on the healing ability that's been placed in them. Our bodies have innate recuperative powers that are inherent. As long as that healing power is expressing itself at full capacity, the body can heal itself. But this is not what people are taught to rely upon.

They're taught to rely on drugs and surgery and to be reactive, to put their body's health in the hands of so-called "qualified experts."

The people who show up at my office typically arrive taking six to eight medications per day, which is what the average American consumes. According to the Center for Disease Control, the average sixty-five-year-old can be taking up to thirteen medications. Clearly, something is not working. People are going to doctors for pain management, but instead are being prescribed drugs, which ultimately create more pain and complicate health issues. Using more drugs is like pouring kerosene on a fire.

Our clinical complaints range from autoimmune diseases, multiple sclerosis, rheumatoid arthritis, lupus, neck pain, back pain, asthma, and allergies to big-time offenders such as diabetes, cancer, heart disease, thyroid issues and strokes. Disease, in general, is more rampant than ever before. In fact, in 2008, Americans were ranked as one of the sickest industrialized nations in the world, as well as the most obese and overweight country in the world. We also have more degenerative disease than any other industrialized country along with the highest rate of depression. In a recent comparison with other countries, the United States ranked at the bottom regarding several health categories. More specifically, the ranking of the U.S. with thirteen other top industrialized nations on various indicators was:

- Thirteenth (last) for low birth-weight percentages.

- Thirteenth for neonatal mortality and overall infant mortality.

- Eleventh for post neonatal mortality.

- Eleventh for life expectancy at one year for females, twelfth for males.

- Tenth for life expectancy at fifteen years for females, twelfth for males.

- Tenth for life expectancy at forty years for females, ninth for males.

- Seventh for life expectancy at sixty-five years for females, seventh for males.

- Third for life expectancy at eighty years for females, third for males.

- Tenth for age-adjusted mortality.

- Thirteenth for years of potential life lost (excluding external causes).

New research shows that the estimated total number of deaths inadvertently induced by a physician or surgeon or by medical treatment or diagnostic procedures annually in the United States is between 783,936 and 999,936. From these updated numbers it becomes evident that our conventional, modern medical system is itself the leading cause of death and injury in the United States. (approximately 699,697 Americans died of heart disease in 2001 and 553,251 died of cancer. These numbers are derived from the total deaths directly attributed to adverse drug reactions, medical error, bedsores, infections, malnutrition in hospitals, outpatients, unnecessary procedures, and those related to surgery. When the number one killer in a society is the health-care system, to not address this major shortcoming is a serious issue. It's a failed system in need of immediate attention and urgent repair.

More on the state of our 'sick care' system:

- One in three Americans will have cancer in their lifetime

- One in eight women will be diagnosed with breast cancer

- Heart disease kills more women than breast cancer

- One and a half million Americans have heart attacks every year—500,000 of them die

- One million new cases of diabetes reported per year

- Thirty-three million Americans suffer from arthritis

- Eighteen percent of Americans have hypertension

- One in five Americans have anxiety or depression disorder

- With more than 7,000 new cases every year, cancer kills more children than any other disease

- One out of two children will develop heart disease

- Two in five American children are obese

- One out of twelve children will develop diabetes

- By the age of three, children have fatty deposits in their arteries

- By age twelve, 70 percent of American children are in the early stages of hardening of the arteries

- Seven to 10 percent of school-age children are diagnosed with Attention Deficit disorder (ADD/ADHD).

Denis Cortese, M.D., the Mayo Clinic's president and chief executive officer, had the following to say in a recent interview: "To the extent that people say our health-care system is broken, I would reject that as a too-simple thought. There is no system. So let's design one. The fatal problem that all of our people in Washington have—and many people have in the country: They've come to believe that the system is "broken." That's like saying, "I've got a broken car." And you're going to go out and you're going to fix it. And you go in the garage and you find out, "Oh, I forgot. I don't have a car." You can't fix something that doesn't exist. Nobody ever designed this to be a system. Nobody's ever sat down to say here's where we want to be in the future. That's what we're trying to do. We're trying to get across the message that we've got things that aren't working. Yes, we have a catastrophe coming at us."

Clearly, nothing that people are currently doing for their health outside the realm of natural healing is working, with the exception of emergency and crisis medical intervention. Drugs and surgery are clearly not working to produce health and wellness. Based on the argument that we have more drugs and surgery than any other country, we should be the healthiest country in the world. But we're not. This is happening because the only people who are teaching the public about health are the drug companies. These companies have a monopoly on the psyche of America. People's perception, their understanding of the concept of health, is that if you have a problem, you take a drug. There's a pill, potion, lotion, spoonful-of-medicine mentality that makes people think drugs will cure any ailment. If you're depressed, you take this pill. If you have a stomach ache, you take that pill. If you have asthma or allergies, you take this type of medication. If you have diabetes, you take that type of medication. If you have high cholesterol or high blood pressure, you take these medications. Now take this pill to counteract the effects of the other medications. This is what is happening in our country. The drug companies are teaching the public that if you have a problem, the solution comes in a pill bottle.

In November 2007, the FDA released a sixty-page report titled "FDA Science and Mission at Risk." In this report, the agency admitted that it lacked the competency and capacity to keep up with scientific advances. The FDA now admits that Americans are suffering and dying because the FDA does not have the scientific ability to evaluate claims or to ascertain whether new drugs are safe or effective.

A BRIEF HISTORY OF MEDICINE

The history of pharmaceutical misinformation can be traced to the Rockefellers and the Carnegies at the turn of the nineteenth century. That's who started pumping tons of money into the drug industry. They saw a tremendous opportunity to make lots of money, so they started funding medical schools. At that point in time, medical schools were designed to just teach surgery. The Rockefellers and Carnegies introduced the drug industry because they knew that by doing so they could expand and glean huge profits. That's when the drug era really began. Because of the funding, they were able to market on a tremendous level. In fact, today marketing budgets are up to billions of dollars, and the drug companies can reach billions of people with their message. They have penetrated the subconscious of the American culture to the point where they control the thinking and health-care decisions of almost all Americans. The author of a recent Journal of the American Medical Association report is Dr. Barbara Starfield of the Johns Hopkins School of Hygiene and Public Health. She shockingly describes that the problem is the "U.S. health-care system itself, and not lifestyle or a lack of technology that is actually the major contributor to our low rankings and our poor health."

THE COST OF BAD "HEALTH" CARE

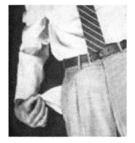

A recent study by Harvard University researchers found that 50 percent of all bankruptcy filings were partly the result of medical expenses. The average out-of-pocket medical debt for those who filed for bankruptcy was $12,000. The study noted that 68 percent of those who filed for bankruptcy had health insurance. Every thirty seconds in the United States someone files for bankruptcy in the aftermath of a serious health problem. A new survey shows that more than 25 percent said that housing problems resulted from medical debt, including the inability to make rent or mortgage payments and the development of bad credit ratings. About 1.5 million families lose their homes to foreclosure every year due to unaffordable medical costs. A survey of Iowa consumers found that to cope with rising health insurance costs, 86 percent said they had cut back on how much they could save, and 44 percent said that they had cut back on food and heating expenses. Retiring elderly couples will need $250,000 in savings just to pay for the most basic medical coverage. Many experts believe that this figure is conservative and that $300,000 may be a more realistic number.

Public health advocates believe that if all Americans adopted healthy lifestyles, health-care costs would decrease as people would require less medical care.

THE ALTERNATIVE TO MEDICINE

In my office, we see the results of chiropractic care, because we begin with the understanding that the body has an inherent wisdom and self-recuperative power that resides within every single cell at every level. It forms when a sperm and an egg come together, at conception. There is a miracle that happens when God breathes life into that cell. There's a cell division process that begins, and from that point forward, that intelligence develops that single cell into a human being over nine months. We'll come back to this, but the thing running this entire process is the nervous system, which is really at the core of this entire book and the core of being healthy. It's the backbone to true health, healing, and well-being.

That health and that healing intelligence never leave the body. Through nine months of development, and even when the child is born, that innate healing recuperative power resides within every cell of the body. And as long as that healing power can express itself, we have the ability to live healthy, drug-free, surgery-free lives from cradle to grave—to at least 120 years of good healthy living, as science and biblical knowledge promise us.

The process of reeducation is to first and foremost show people the amazing innate healing power that resides within the body. This is something that we can put our faith in. It's something that we really, truly can rely upon to get our bodies well. So the main process in reeducating people is giving them the understanding that there is a primary system inside the human body. There are many organs inside your body, but there's only one that controls every single part, every function: the nervous system. It controls, coordinates, harmonizes, and governs all healing. It runs everything, and as long as it's working properly, the body has an innate ability to express optimal health and wellness. When the system works at its peak, you can then express full human potential and perform at your intellectual, physical, mental, and emotional best. When people understand that, and they have confidence, faith, and trust in this concept and nervous system, then they can truly start making the shift into allowing their bodies to heal normally, properly, and on their own.

Shifting the paradigm is all about education. Our patients begin to understand that it is normal, not abnormal, for people to be well. We provide people with empowering resources and information, continuously reinforce it, and daily educate them with the message. In my office, we write newsletters. We have classes and workshops. We give people tools and programs that we hope will change their outlook and shift their paradigm back to what it was before the drug companies got to it. We aim to replace the massive amounts of misinformation and empower the public with the truth. And this book is one of the places to start.

> *"The person who takes medicine must recover twice, once from the disease and once from the medicine."*
> *William Osler, M.D.*

After years and years of drug usage and surgeries, of their bodies breaking down, people walk into my office and we explain to them that there's a process of healing. We need to get the neurological system functioning properly so it can bring back life, health, and rejuvenation to every cell in the body. There is a process, like there is a process to reach sickness. All kinds of symptoms were manifested along that path. In the same light, if someone wants to go back to where they came from, to true optimal health and healing, some may have to retrace that path for their bodies to heal.

This is not easy for some people. They have to go through pain again, maybe through headaches, through manifestations of different symptoms, but this is part of the healing process. It's not unusual to not want to have to go through pain again. People often want to take a pill and be done with it; they want a quick fix because we live in a quick-fix society. But healing properly comes from what we call "above-down-inside-out," which means it comes from the nervous system and the brain, through the spine, and out to the organs of the body. Unfortunately, it takes time. It's different for everybody. It depends upon how long the sickness has been there, how long the person has been struggling, and how far the body has degenerated. It depends upon age, the number of traumas, the number of drugs taken, and the number of emotional, chemical, physical, mental, and spiritual traumas in a lifetime. All these are calculated and figured into the equation, into the formula of healing. For children, it's a lot faster, obviously. The earlier we can get into that process, the faster it's going to happen. For some people, it can be a couple of days or weeks, and for some people it can take years. Some must go through an enormous amount of symptomology as they retrace that path of sickness and disease. Then again, some people experience no symptoms at all, and some people experience immediate relief. However, there is one single, expected result: healing

ONE CAUSE, ONE CURE

All disease, all sickness, all pain, and all suffering within the human body come from interference. That is, interference to the innate expression of optimal health and healing or the God-given healing potential innately resident in your own body. You might ask how that can be interfered with, but it is interfered with chemically, emotionally, or physically every day in all sorts of ways. When the interference is lessened, a person can express optimal health and healing. It's just like taking your foot off a garden hose. If the hose is going to a garden bed, fertilizing and watering, bringing nutrients and nourishment, and you have your foot on it, the nutrition will not be able to get to where it is supposed to, and the plants will die. It doesn't matter how good the soil is or how much sunshine those plants are getting. A vital element of nourishment is missing. It's the same with your body. When you remove the interference, the body naturally begins to express this healing potential. It was there all along; the body just needed to have the interference removed. Overall, healing the body has more to do with what you need to stop doing to the body, than what you need to do or give to the body.

Remember, the healing process occurs through only one system of the body: the nervous system. And in the nervous system, there is one organ that controls every single aspect of healing: the brain. The heart doesn't control the body. The liver doesn't. The stomach doesn't. It's the brain, which is included in the central nervous system. The spine is the connection between the brain and the organs of the body; messages from the brain flow through the spine and out through the nerves into every single organ of the body. If unblocked, this produces life, health, and healing.

There are four essentials to life, healing, optimal health expression, and longevity: food, water, air, and nerve supply. But which is the most important? Well, you can go at least forty days without food. Water, you can go several days without. Air, you can go maybe a few minutes. But we know that if you disturb brain-body communication, you'll have a problem within milliseconds. Out of the four, a healthy nerve supply certainly is the most important. All health and healing comes through the nervous system; the system that controls and regulates every cell and every function of your body.

What I would like you to take away from this book, more than anything else, is hope – hope that as long as this healing power can flow with no interference, be it chemical, emotional, or physical, your body can heal any disease or sickness and end any pain. I want you to know that you can overcome any obstacle or challenge you might have in your health and well-being. I've seen every disease you can name walk through my clinic door and have watched the body recover and heal, but only after the patient took the first step and only after the interference was removed.

CHAPTER TWO

TRADITIONAL MEDICINE: THE TRUTH REVEALED

"The cause of most disease is in the poisonous drugs physicians superstitiously give in order to effect a cure."

–Charles E. Page, M.D.

"As a retired physician, I can honestly say that unless you are in a serious accident, your best chance of living to a ripe old age is to avoid doctors and hospitals and learn nutrition, herbal medicine, and other forms of natural medicine. Almost all drugs are toxic and are designed only to treat symptoms and not to cure anyone. Vaccines are highly dangerous, have never been adequately studied or proven to be effective, and have a poor risk/reward ratio. Most surgery is unnecessary, and most textbooks of medicine are inaccurate and deceptive. Almost every disease is said to be idiopathic (without known cause) or genetic, although this is untrue. In short, our mainstream medical system is hopelessly inept and/or corrupt. The treatment of cancer and degenerative diseases is a national scandal. The sooner you learn this, the better off you will be."   –Dr. Allan Greenberg, M.D.

lead to all sorts of health concerns: high blood pressure, heart disease, obesity, and high cholesterol.

So as you can see, all kinds of things happen as a result of stress. Your doctor is going to want to treat your cholesterol, diabetes, etc., but he's not going to treat you for the stress that caused the problems. Most doctors try to change these natural consequences of living in a stressful environment, but no pill, potion, lotion, or spoonful of medicine can ever change the stress.

The bottom line is this: Medicine looks at the effects and then treats or covers up the symptoms. While the fire alarm is going off and the building is burning down, doctors reach up into the fire alarm and pull the battery out so they don't have to hear the noise. Chiropractors look to the cause.

EMERGENCY MEDICINE

This is not to say that traditional medicine doesn't have its uses. Thank God for drugs and surgery in emergency crisis intervention. However, medical experts tell us that emergency medicine and crisis care are needed in perhaps 0.5 to 1 percent of medically related health problems. And in those cases, thank God we have the best emergency care in the world, but we have to learn how and when to use it. One thing we know, as proven by hundreds of research studies: hospitals are really the best place to go if you want to die or get a new infection.

The smartest thing you can do as a health-care consumer is to understand how and when to use drugs, surgery, emergency care, and the tests doctors give you. I have patients who come to my office with 201 cholesterol levels (under 200 is considered medically 'normal') and they have "high" written on their lab tests, and their doctors are recommending Lipitor or some type of statin/cholesterol lowering drug. These people deserve to understand what a 201 cholesterol level means and how to interpret it. Many medical tests give a false positive reading, which means they are inaccurate.

In fact, many of the medical tests are turning out to be extremely dangerous. There's a lot of talk in the scientific community regarding the issue of mammograms and how they possibly could be causing breast cancer. The belief has been that women could be saved from breast cancer by shooting radiation through their breasts every year. However, the breast is very sensitive tissue, and radiating this tissue regularly can create cancer. There's a time and a place to get medical tests, but make sure you understand the ramifications and what the information means. Then decide what to do with that information.

Again, thank God for drugs and surgery in heath emergencies. I know that lives have been saved because drugs and surgery were available—but both must be used intelligently. A drug can be a lifelong necessity if an organ has been removed and is not available to function. But drugs and surgery in the long term will generally do nothing but destroy the human body. If you're going to be well, long term, you must adopt healthy lifestyle practices, or else your body will continue to rely upon drugs and surgery. If you keep taking drugs, your doctor will probably want you to stay on them long term.

People should utilize emergency care wisely and prudently. What constitutes an emergency? Obvious examples include: broken bones, bleeding arteries; a case of a child running a fever who is listless, dulleyed, not moving, or extremely lethargic – these are emergencies. My hope for everybody who is reading this book is to have a team of health-care providers and regular checkups. For the most part, I think common sense tells us what's an emergency and what is not.

WHY DRUGS?

Clinical statistics provide interesting discussions. One thing you'll see with drug companies is that they often do their own drug trials and publish the literature available on the drug themselves! An inherent conflict of interest exists there. When you see on TV that a drug has been shown to be safe and effective, often the claim is based on selective and/or manipulated statistics and not factual data derived from independent, unbiased research. For instance, it's now been shown that walking three times a week for thirty minutes could possibly work better than a well known antidepressant, one which earns multibillion-dollar annual sales. Nobody knew that because the statistics were skewed. They were manipulated to represent something different than they really demonstrated.

John Abramson, M.D., points out in his book, *Overdosed America*, that a 2002 article in the Journal of the American Medical Association showed that "59 percent of the experts who write the clinical guidelines that define good medical care (the standards to which doctors are often held in malpractice) have direct financial ties to the companies whose products are being evaluated." If doctors choose to ignore guidelines, they risk their reputations, their standing in the medical community, and being charged with malpractice.

Drugs never get to the cause of the problem because their nature is to mask symptoms, and that is inherently what is wrong with our "health-care system." In reality, it's a "sick and disease care" system.

Drugs will not get rid of the cause of your headache, your high blood pressure, your high cholesterol, your stomach ache, your asthma or your allergies; drugs just make you feel more comfortable and alter your body chemistry. They reduce your symptoms while, in fact, your body is slowly dying because the cells are now being poisoned and the root cause of your problem has not been removed. Cancer treatments are a perfect example of this. It is estimated that chemotherapy is "effective" in treating only about 2 to 4 percent of cancers, yet $8 billion is spent on this form of treatment each year. Have you ever wondered why is it that we spend billions on treatment and research of cancer, yet cancer rates continue to rise? For instance, in 1973, two out of ten people would develop cancer; today, six out ten people develop some form of cancer. Research shows that mainstream cancer treatments are actually responsible for creating secondary cancers. Many drugs cause cancer as well as other diseases. Here are some examples:

- **Cholesterol medication** – Recently shown to cause an increase in cancer mortality (www.nejm.org.)

- **Arthritis drugs (Tumor Necrosis Factor [TNF] Blockers)** – Causing cancers in children and young adults (WebMD Health News, 2008).

- **Breast cancer drugs** – Shown to cause uterine cancer (International Journal of Gynecological Cancer, 2007).

- **ADD/ADHD drugs** – Cytogenic (chromosomal) damage connection shown (Cancer Letters Volume 230, Issue 2, 18 December 2005).

It's very simple: Put any chemical into your body, and it causes damage. If your body can't heal the damage, you accumulate damage. As damage spreads without healing, this is called disease. If we want to discuss disease, then we must address prevention. Prevention is the cure for cancer or any other disease. We have to try to stop causing it, then we won't have to fight it or treat it (more on this later).

Why is it that so many Americans are taking so many drugs? If we weren't being marketed to, would human beings want to get well without drugs and surgery? If you were sick and suffering and you knew there was a natural, effective way to get well, one that might take a little time, but was safe, gentle and nontoxic, I believe that it would be human nature to naturally gravitate toward that way of healing. Everybody would want that! It's counterintuitive to think that people would want to take a drug. This is why drug companies have to spend billions upon billions of dollars brainwashing—not educating, but brainwashing—Americans to think that drug therapy is the way to take care of their health. Next time you're watching T.V., ask yourself, " how many drug commercials are there per hour?"

Innately, we want natural cures. We want our bodies to heal the way God designed them to heal. However, drug companies are such a powerful marketing force that they have educated Americans for three generations – us, our parents, and grandparents – so well, so effectively and efficiently, that our first nature by default is drug therapy. It's the number one choice when it comes to health care. Someone's sick, and his doctor prescribes a drug just like that. Someone's in pain, and the doctor instantly thinks of surgery. Drug companies have done this to us, and as a result, it seems they're not only manipulating patients, they are also getting the patients to manipulate their doctors. The phrase heard in so many commercials, "Ask your doctor about...," exemplifies this. Pharmaceutical companies spend more than $16 billion each year promoting prescription drugs in the United States. These campaigns are designed to effectively alter the prescribing behavior of your doctor to make sure that the pharmaceutical company's drug is doctor-recommended.

DOCTORS ARE GOOD PEOPLE

Medical doctors don't go to school to hurt people. In fact, I have several doctors of mainstream medicine in my own family. They have great hearts, they're very compassionate, and they genuinely want to serve humanity. But they also have become victims of a system not controlled by them. The medical/disease-care system in our country is controlled by pharmaceutical companies, so when people see advertisements on TV they go to the doctors demanding medications they may not need, for conditions they may not even have. Pharmaceutical representatives educate doctors, and even though the doctors want to help people, they're trapped in this system. Doctors may be smart and nice people, but for most, they no longer control their own decision-making process.

Japan, Sweden, France and Italy consistently rank as the healthiest countries in the world, and if you look at their lifestyle, their life choices, you can see what the difference is. There's a lot less stress, emotionally, chemically and physically. People move their bodies more, for instance, in Japan and Sweden. In Sweden, people are riding bikes everywhere, walking everywhere; they move their bodies on a daily basis. The food and water are less contaminated with pollution and chemicals. Livestock has less hormones, and vegetation less pesticides. Emotional, chemical and physical interferences are far fewer, so these populations are much healthier and happier with a much higher quality of life.

The healthiest countries do not have the psychological saturation of Big Pharma telling them to take drugs. Patients from around the world have commented on the insanity of how many medications Americans take.

When Americans come home from work, we have fifty drug commercials coming at us in thirty minutes telling us which drug to pop. The healthiest countries in the world do not have mass media marketing to them every day to take drugs and submit to surgery. Both are a last option, if an option at all, in these countries. Most of them are taking zero medications, and I believe that's one of the main reasons for their incredible health profile.

SMART MINDS, POOR BODIES

A major reason Americans choose these methods is that some of the brightest people on the planet run this incredibly efficient marketing machine. They know exactly how to penetrate the human psyche. Have you ever noticed how they color pills—the purple pill, the orange pill, the yellow pill? Marketing is fashioned to engage and stimulate certain parts of the brain just to make the product seem enticing.

We live in a quick-fix society. Americans love instant results and gratification, and the drug culture fits right into this fast-track society. Take a look at Botox. Botox, as in botulism, is one of the deadliest naturally occurring toxins. And yet, marketing and pop culture have convinced people that injecting it into their faces to get rid of wrinkles is a good idea. There's no explanation for it other than vanity, and there's no outcome other than sickness for the patient and profit for the company that sold it.

The following is an excerpt from *The Wellness Revolution* by economist Paul Zane Pilzer:

> *"Treating the symptoms of disease rather than preventing disease is more profitable for medical companies; to research and develop products that create customers for life is the goal. How economics perpetuates sickness: just as with consumers, physicians are the target market of the medical and pharmaceutical companies. Patients receive the drug or treatment that is most profitable for the supplier of the treatment, the health insurance company, and, in some cases, even individual physicians. This may or may not represent the best medical treatment available. In the United States, doctors typically prescribe completely different treatments for the same ailment depending on which drug company has a dominant market share in their region. Medical technology and pharmaceuticals change so fast today that what physicians learn at medical school is often outdated by the time they graduate. In practice, doctors learn about the drugs and treatments from a special type of salesperson, called a detail person in the medical industry. Detail person is actually a euphemism for "a very attractive, highly paid young person of the opposite sex." Detail people are lavishly paid. And they handsomely reward the physicians and their staff in proportion to the amount of prescriptions they write for the company's products. Physicians and their families receive expensive dinners, cruises, and tax-free trips to resorts, where they "learn" more about such products at taxpayers' expense."*

CHAPTER THREE

WELLNESS AS
THE ANSWER

"When the solution is simple, God is answering."
—*Albert Einstein*

According to the World Health Organization, "health is more than the absence of disease. Health is a state of optimal well-being." Optimal well-being is a concept of health that goes beyond the curing of illness to one of experiencing wellness. Many of us have been brought up to believe that our health depends solely on the quality of the health care we receive or we are healthy if we have no symptoms. The truth is, your health is your responsibility. If you are going to be well, truly well, you must be proactive.

Isn't it funny how the practice of good spinal health, maintaining excellent nerve function, nutrition, detoxification, exercise, and vitamin supplements, which are all vital to great health and well-being, are called alternative medicine? Wellness practices should be considered primary health care. Traditional medicine is emergency, urgent crisis care, involving drugs and surgery; it is not health care. This should really be called the alternative. The alternative to health, vitality and well-being is lying in a hospital following a trauma or hooked up to an I.V. drip as a scalpel cuts open your abdomen to remove a cancerous lesion. That's the alternative.

More than ever, people are sick of being on medications. They don't want to be asking, "Doctor, why am I forty-five years old and waking up every day with pain all over my body, shooting down my legs and arms? I have headaches every day. I have blurry vision. I have ringing in my ears. I have asthma. I have allergies. I have diabetes. I have no energy. I have fibromyalgia and chronic fatigue. I feel like I'm ninety years old. What is wrong with me?" And they don't want another doctor to say, "Well, take this drug, and give me a call in six weeks. If it hasn't kicked in and if you're still alive, then you can come back and we can give you a different medication and see if that drug works." This is ultimately not what people really want. People want to know the cause. They want to know what's wrong with them. And they want to know how to get better.

This is the doctor of the future: Someone who can find out exactly what's wrong with people and help them get well and stay that way as long as possible, with as little investment in time and money as possible. That's what people want. They simply want results. They don't want their problems covered up, because that means they're just going to get sicker. People are getting wiser today. Despite all the pharmaceutical brain-washing and so-called education, they still understand that their bodies will only get sicker if the cause of the problem isn't treated. Many people walk into my clinic putting their faith and confidence in me to get their life and their health back. They walk in believing they're going to experience changes and that their pain or disease won't be covered up but rather will be removed. They really believe this. They know if we can get to the cause of the problem and remove the interference, whether physical, chemical, or emotional, they're going to receive and achieve extraordinary health.

"The doctor of the future will give no medicine, but will interest his patients in diet and in the cause and prevention of disease; and in the care of the human frame." Thomas Edison

People want a doctor who looks at the whole person. They want someone who looks to the causes of their problems in a holistic, wellness-oriented way and then offers a way to achieve optimal health and well-being. People want a doctor who's going to equip them with all the resources and knowledge to begin making the shift in their lifestyle that will produce health in the long term. These people don't want a quick fix but a lifestyle that will produce lasting health and healing. They're looking for a doctor to educate them on the culture of health. That's what the doctor of the future does, and what I've created in my office. We give people stress and time management tips. We discuss all this in the office and also run wellness workshops which teach optimal lifestyle habits and strategies.

Medicine is catching on to this and trying to change its stripes. Fortunately, the industry has started trying to give people what they're looking for. In my town, for instance, a lot of the medical doctors offer nutrition or exercise tips. They're trying to offer one piece of the puzzle. In our office, we put all the pieces together and connect them. This is what the doctor of the future will do: bring it all together with an understanding and the ability to communicate that the nervous system—the spine—is the core of a healthy lifestyle. Eating properly, thinking properly, and moving properly are all the right decisions, coordinated by the nervous system, with the effect of good health.

Even though medicine is trying to move toward these options, often it falls short. Doctors of chiropractic, however, bring together all of the components of a healthy nervous system and brain-body connection.

I find it interesting that in many villages in China, and throughout Asia, the doctor only gets paid when the patient is well. When the patient falls ill, the doctor's compensation comes to a halt. This system definitely provides a strong motivating force for the doctor to produce results!

VITAL REPORT ON CANCER
RECENTLY RELEASED

"The Conception of Wellness," a new Harvard Health Publications wellness study by Hillary M. Wright, reports a finding by the American Institute for Cancer Research (AICR) that 50 percent of Americans think preventing cancer is either impossible or highly unlikely. Only 49 percent were aware that diets low in fruits and vegetables increase cancer risk. Only 46 percent cited obesity as a risk factor for cancer. Only 37 percent knew of alcohol's link to cancer. Only 36 percent were aware of the link between diets high in red meat – particularly processed meat – and cancer.

The World Cancer Research Fund (WCRF) says about one third of cancers worldwide could be avoided through diet and activity. The report, called "Food, Nutrition, Physical Activity and the Prevention of Cancer: A Global Perspective," took five years to complete and was based on more than 7,000 scientific studies. It is the most comprehensive review ever published of the science linking cancer risk to diet, physical activity and weight.

Report recommendations:

- Be as lean as possible within your normal body weight range.

- Be physically active as part of everyday life.

- Limit calorie-dense food you eat (those high in fat and sugar) and avoid sugary drinks.

- Eat mostly foods of plant origin – fruits, vegetables, and whole grains.

- Limit intake of red meat (beef, pork and lamb) and avoid processed meats, such as bacon, sausage, bologna, ham and salami.

- Limit your intake of alcoholic beverages.

- Limit your salt intake.

Other important points:

- Try to meet your nutritional needs through diet alone.

- Mothers should breast feed their babies as it lowers the risk of breast cancer and reduces their child's risk of obesity later in life.

- Cancer survivors should be encouraged to follow the report's recommendations for cancer prevention and seek the advice of a trained nutrition professional.

The report found convincing evidence for a link between cancer and the following lifestyle situations:

Excess weight: especially abdominal fat, increased the risk of post-menopausal breast cancer, and cancers of the colon, pancreas, kidney, endometrium, and esophagus. Those who are obese have raised levels of numerous cancer-promoting hormones and other factors. In fact, excess weight is now second only to cigarette smoking as a preventable cause of cancer.

Physical activity: All forms of activity can protect against colon cancer and probably protect against post-menopausal breast cancer and endometrial cancer. Active people have healthier levels of circulating hormones and may be able to eat more without gaining weight.

Red meat consumption: We have stronger evidence now than in 1997 (when the report was last compiled) that high intakes of red and processed meats – especially those preserved with smoking, curing or salt – increase the risk of colorectal cancer.

Alcohol consumption: even moderate, may increase risk of cancers of the head and neck, esophagus, colorectum (in men), and breast. It also is considered a probable cause of liver cancer and colorectal cancer in women.

Plant foods: The report strongly encourages eating mostly plant foods due to their "probable" protective effect against cancers of the digestive tract, lung and prostate, and known connection to successful weight loss.

What are your best bets for staying cancer-free per the report:

- Make weight loss a priority by watching portions, avoiding sugary drinks, and significantly limiting "fast foods" and other foods high in fat and sugar.

- Aim for at least five servings of fruits and vegetables daily.

- Aim for thirty minutes of aerobic activity daily, either at once or in short spurts, with a long-term goal of sixty minutes of activity most days. Limit red meat to eighteen ounces or less per week, and avoid processed meats.

- Drink alcohol in moderation, if at all.

Wellness care begins the first day of life. It actually begins before conception. In our office, we teach future moms and dads how to get their bodies healthy and whole prior to conceiving a child. We begin right from the beginning of life. I go to homes, I go to hospitals, and I check the babies at birth. I check their spines, especially the atlas (upper neck region) at the beginning. Health begins with natural childbirth, a home delivery or birthing center with a midwife. When this is possible, I feel it is the best option. Birthing centers and midwives are highly trained and qualified to deliver babies and understand how to deal with emergencies and work with emergency personnel. Health also begins with breastfeeding or feeding non-sugar-laden formulas. Most of the formulas available are loaded with corn starches, corn syrup, and soy, as well as neurotoxins – all kinds of junk that is horrible for the developing child. Breast feeding (when possible) is an essential component to producing a healthy child and setting that child up for a lifetime of optimal performance and health. I teach parents how to get their child moving and keep them away from TV.

According to the Academy of Physicians and Surgeons, children under the age of two should avoid watching television. It destroys neurological development. This is how you raise a healthy family and healthy children. This is what wellness care means when developing a healthy family. You should start as soon as possible. The most critical component is making sure the nervous system is healthy right at the beginning of life—not only making sure the two parents have healthy brain-body connections and neurology and a minimal amount of subluxation/neurological interference (preconception, ideally), but also that the child has his or her backbone of health working properly.

> *"For every drug that benefits a patient, there is a natural substance that can achieve the same effect."* — *Pfeiffer's Law*

Instead of asking why you should start a wellness program, the question you should be asking is why shouldn't you. Why wouldn't you want to be well and perform at your best? Why wouldn't you want to a part of the culture of health? Why would you not avoid taking drugs? Would you want to get surgery if you didn't have to?

What are some of the things that you want to do in your life? How long do you want to live? Where do you want to go? What are the dreams you have? The aspirations? Do you want to enjoy your children, your grandchildren, and your great-grandchildren? What is the juice you want to squeeze out of life? What do you want to do with this lifetime God has given you? What are the things you want to do financially, relationship-wise, emotionally, and physically?

Without health, wellness, and energy, without having a healthy body and a healthy mind, you can't do any of them. They're all worthless without health. When you have health and wellness, when you're emotionally, mentally, and physically strong and healthy, life takes on a whole different meaning. You perceive life differently. Every part of life expresses itself better, more fully, and you become more fulfilled—you and your children. Drugs blur and distort your perception and experience of life. They blur and distort your mental and emotional interpretation of the events in your life.

When children are healthier they can think better, they can get better grades, they behave better, and they focus better. They don't need to go onto ADD and ADHD drugs. They get along with their peers better. They can contribute more to the world. And overall, more than anything, they can serve their creator on a higher level, and thus can serve their brothers and sisters on a higher level. And by doing that, they can contribute to this planet, to humanity, on a greater level and leave a powerful legacy, if that's what they choose to do.

IS IT WORTH THE COST?

People often ask me how much a healthy life like this costs. All I can tell them is that relative to the cost of sickness, it's practically free. Right now, at a bare minimum, the current cost of having heart disease is $150,000 to $160,000 in medical bills. Cancer runs the average patient around $100,000, though some cancer treatments range between $10,000 and $20,000 per month. Even the best insurances in the world might deny your claim, and you end up bankrupt.

Right now, conventional wisdom claims medical bills cause 50 percent of all bankruptcy in America, and most of these people had "good" insurance. For instance, I had a gentleman come to my office the day after he went to the hospital with a heart problem. His heart was beating out of control, and so he went to the doctor to be admitted and he came out with a $21,000 bill. His heart problem was still there; it was still racing. After one adjustment at my office, his problem was gone.

He now has a $21,000 bill, which, by the way, his insurance will not pay. He could have received wellness care at my office for decades for that amount of money. He is a perfect example that keeping healthy and staying healthy is a lot less expensive than getting sick and going through the medical system. Not only is it more expensive to your bank account, it's more expensive to your loved ones. It's absolutely devastating when a loved one is ill, and it's a struggle to have to take care of a sick person. The costs are enormous, not only financially, but also emotionally and physically. Everybody ages, everybody gets stressed out. There is no doubt about it: Staying healthy is a lot easier and less expensive.

A lot of people complain that organic fruits and vegetables cost too much, that gym memberships cost too much, that eating healthy takes too much time, and that regular wellness chiropractic care is too much of an expense. I could guarantee you that staying healthy and maintaining your health is a lot less expensive than waiting until you're sick and trying to dig yourself out of a hole with drugs and surgery. Case in point: I have observed that almost all traffic injuries and fatalities are caused by someone who is either under the influence, taking a pharmaceutical drug, or in a lot of pain with a lot of health problems – perhaps blocked arteries. Their brains are not getting oxygenated.

How many things can go wrong when we don't feel good mentally, emotionally, and physically? We're much more prone to injuries from falling or slipping. Our immune systems are compromised. These costs far exceed the costs of staying well and maintaining health and well-being.

H.S.A.

A health savings account (H.S.A.) is a wonderful invention. It hasn't been around for long, but people are beginning to learn more about it every day. An H.S.A. is basically a way for you to hold on to your own health-care dollars. Instead of sending them off to some faceless insurance company, you fund your own health insurance. You put your own money in, then you can self-direct it. It's almost like an I.R.A. in that you can take that health savings account and invest it wherever you'd like. Plus, you usually earn about 5 or 7 percent interest on your own money. It's your money, and in most cases, it's tax-free. So, when you take that money out you can use it for whatever you want.

A lot of people who come into my office have a massage therapist, nutritionist, chiropractor, acupuncturist, and dentist. They have formed their own health team, which most of the time their insurance companies will either not pay for, or will give them a hard time about reimbursing. If you set up one of these, you can use your money in your HSA to pay for these services, and it's all tax-deductible because it's going toward your health care. It's very versatile, so if you just want it to build up for five or ten years, that's fine. The beauty of it is that you have control of your health-care dollars. You appropriate the funds to whatever practitioner you want to visit. It's the definition of health-care freedom.

My own preference is to have a high-deductible catastrophic insurance policy on top of the H.S.A. In the case of a major health emergency, your provider will pay for the hospital care, emergency surgery, etc. I've seen these policies as cheap as seventy dollars a month, up to two hundred dollars per month per family. The catastrophic policy is a cheap form of insurance to cover you only in emergencies.

THREE PILLARS OF WELLNESS

"My fellow medical doctors, look well to the spine for the cause of disease, for it is requisite in the causation of disease."
-Hippocrates, 300 BC (the father of modern medicine)

Some people are afraid to go to a doctor who does not hold a medical degree. Their doctor may have communicated to them in such a way that surgery and drugs seem to be the only option. The important thing to remember here is, first of all, chiropractors do have doctorate degrees. They learn about the body, its functions and vulnerabilities, just as medical physicians do. They are considered primary-care doctors in all fifty states and many foreign countries. However, they are not influenced by Big Pharma. They do not go to schools that are influenced by Big Pharma. Chiropractors are not exposed to the persuasive drug sales representatives who permeate mainstream medicine. Therefore, it makes sense that they are open to alternatives to drugs and surgery.

The qualifications of a licensed chiropractor include a degree from an accredited, licensed chiropractic college. They then sit for a state board and are licensed through this process. The qualifications in the state of Florida where I practice are a four-year undergraduate degree, four years of chiropractic school, and then an internship. Many chiropractors like myself have a degree in nutrition. I have a four-year science degree in nutrition from the University of Florida, which I use to augment my practice and care for my patients. Many wellness chiropractors do post-graduate studies in bio-structural spinal correction, nutrition, sports fitness and exercise physiology, neurology, and lifestyle coaching.

You should expect several things from a chiropractor. First, wellness chiropractors like me are extraordinarily good at making sure they optimize first and foremost the brain-body connection. By working with the spine and nervous system, we optimize the expression of brain-body communication, thus enhancing overall human performance. We do this by making sure the spine has all the normal curves. We look for and reduce vertebral subluxation. A vertebral subluxation is when bones of the spinal column are out of alignment, causing interference in this communication. This is what my dad had for years following his head trauma, resulting in his debilitating migraines.

There are twenty-four moveable bones in the spine, plus the sacrum and the coccyx. When these bones shift because of stress or a fall, slip, or injury, sleeping the wrong way, a car accident, a repetitive injury, or just sitting all day working on a computer the spine moves out of alignment. This misalignment can irritate and put pressure directly or indirectly on the spinal cord or the nerves surrounding it. This then electrically short-circuits the neurological system and thereby creates a blockage or interference of the normal expression of healing coming from the brain through the spinal cord and out to the body. A qualified wellness chiropractor is trained to detect and correct subluxations. We're trained to remove this electrical interference with our hands and with instruments. Removing the interference from the brain to the body optimizes the expression of health and healing.

In my office, we use a bio-structural technique to restore normal, natural curves in all regions of the spine: the cervical, thoracic, and lumbar regions. We use diagnostics to make sure that not only is the spine going back to the proper alignment visually, but also electrically the body is functioning better. The types of diagnostics and imaging we use are identical to the technology in the mainstream medical field: X-rays, thermal imaging, surface E.M.G.s, and a number of other examinations.

The second issue we address with our patients is chemical interferences. We address the nutritional aspects. Someone may have been exposed to neurotoxic or biotoxic pathogens. Maybe they've had a mercury exposure or vaccine poisoning. Maybe they've been exposed to a biotoxic mold poisoning or Lyme disease. Maybe they live in a house where toxins are emanating from the carpet, the furniture, the walls and the drywall, or from the wood. There are many kinds of neurotoxins and biotoxins, and even chemicals in food such as hormones, antibiotics, pesticides, fungicides, and herbicides. These go into our tissues.

The third aspect upon which we focus includes emotional, mental, and spiritual interference which we address in lifestyle changes, peace management, and time management through various workshops that we hold in the office.

These are the three primary aspects that most wellness chiropractors are trained to address to optimize the expression of full health and healing. Again, it doesn't matter how sick you've been. When these three pillars of health, wellness, and longevity are addressed, we see extraordinary changes in people's lives.

Everybody can get well and stay well through wellness care. There are different degrees, obviously, because if you've had your chest cut open and surgeons have altered physical components of your heart, there's only a certain level that you can reach in cardiovascular fitness. If you've had a lobe of your lung removed or your thyroid cut out of your body, there's only so far you can go. However, when you remove the interferences from the three pillars, you optimize the full healing potential of your body and reach your full genetic expression. And the great news is that your genetic expression can be changed.

WELLNESS CARE AND GENETIC EXPRESSION

Dr. Bruce Lipton, author of *The Biology of Belief,* states, "Genes can't turn themselves on and off." Something that affects your internal environment has to trigger them. Genes, like a gun, are only dangerous when the trigger is pulled. Some people have a genetic tendency toward heart disease, breast cancer, mental and emotional disorders, etc., but they are not sentenced to get them. Single gene disorders affect less than 2 percent of the population. As it turns out, you are a remarkable, dynamic being capable of programming or reprogramming yourself to be a healthy, creative, purpose-filled, and joyful person. "It's the environment, not the DNA," says Dr. Lipton. "When I provide a healthy environment for my cells (under the microscope), they thrived; when the environment was less than optimal, the cells faltered. When I adjusted the environment, these "sick" cells revitalized. A lot of people say that bad genetics is the cause of their sickness and suffering. We cannot readily change what codes our genetic blueprints, but we can change our minds!"

According to the top genetic scientists in the world, only 3 percent of degenerative disease is genetic. Ninety-seven percent of degenerative disease such as cancer, heart disease, diabetes, stroke, Alzheimer's, Parkinson's, multiple sclerosis, rheumatoid arthritis, lupus, obesity, psoriasis, and other autoimmune diseases, as well as osteoporosis, are preventable. We must understand that we don't just get or "catch" disease; we often have an active role in acquiring disease. We don't just wake up with heart disease or arthrosclerosis; we bring it on ourselves over many years.

For example, there are breast cancer suppressor genes (BRCA1 and BRCA2), and these genes can be turned off and on. BRCA1 and BRCA2 are human genes that belong to a class known as tumor suppressors. In normal cells, BRCA1 and BRCA2 help ensure the stability of the cell's genetic material (DNA) and help prevent uncontrolled cell growth. Mutation of these genes has been linked to the development of hereditary breast and ovarian cancer. For example, if a woman keeps her body lean (with a body mass index under 24), she can decrease the chance of BRCA 1 and 2 mutation and thus prevent the development of breast cancer by at least 65 percent. Scientists have also found an obesity gene that can be turned off and on; it was found as often among the Amish as in the general American population. But the gene isn't expressed in the Amish community. Why? The Amish spend their days planting, farming, working, building – they're constantly moving their bodies. By doing so, they turn off the expression of the obesity gene. On average, a European walks five to seven miles per day. Americans only walk a tenth of a mile per day. That's all the exercise we're getting. We jump in the car and go to the fast-food drive-through. We go to our offices, sit down all day, get back in the car, go back through the drive-through, go into our garage, and sit onto the couch. That's our tenth of a mile right there; that much walking. That's pretty much all we get.

Dr. Dean Ornish is head of the Preventive Medicine Research Institute in Sausalito, Calif. and a well-known author advocating lifestyle changes to improve health. In a small study, the researchers tracked 30 men with low-risk prostate cancer who decided against conventional medical treatment such as surgery and radiation or hormone therapy.

The men underwent three months of major lifestyle changes, including eating a diet rich in fruits, vegetables, whole grains, legumes and soy products, moderate exercise such as walking half an hour a day, and an hour of daily stress management methods including meditation.

As expected, they lost weight, lowered their blood pressure, and saw other health improvements. But the researchers found more profound changes when they compared prostate biopsies taken before and after the lifestyle changes. After only three months, the men had changes in activity in about 500 genes —including 48 that were turned on and 453 genes that were turned off. The activity of disease-preventing genes increased while a number of disease-promoting genes, including those involved in prostate cancer and breast cancer, shut down, according to the study published in the journal *Proceedings of the National Academy of Sciences.*

David Baltimore, former Nobel Prize laureate, says, "The human genes are like the keys on a keyboard and when you walk up to it you can determine the syntax that you're going to be typing on the keyboard." So for example, if I wake up this morning and I grab for the Pop Tarts and the Fruit Loops, I'm going to have a much different biological expression (phenotypic expression, i.e. genes expressed according to lifestyle) than if I consumed an organic vegetable shake.

I personally consume a healthy nutrient-dense shake every morning that has phyto-nutrient rich greens, which aid in destroying cancer cells and also give me amazing energy for four or five hours. It makes my body feel great. Obviously, did I type a different syntax on my "keys?" Yes. And there are mornings I wake up and eat garbage food, too (although not many!). I also know how awful I feel, but no one is perfect.

Many of the individuals in Dr. Ornish's study had histories of rampant disease throughout their family. Excuses like bad genes and hereditary links are no longer valid. You are not the victim of your genetics. Again, David Baltimore said only 3 percent of your genes actually predict whether you're going to develop a degenerative disease: cancer, heart disease, stroke, diabetes, rheumatoid arthritis, auto-immune diseases. That 3 percent includes children born with Down syndrome or muscular dystrophy, and it is important to keep in mind that 97 percent of all diseases are environmentally caused. We now know this through the new field of genetics called epigenetics. We know that it's   the environment that changes the expression of genes (phenotype). Again, the genes are like the keys on a keyboard. The syntax you type into those keys determines the expression or compo-sition. In another way genes are like the trigger on a gun, and the environment determines whether or not the trigger is pulled. If you wake up every morning and drink Yoo-hoo and eat Twinkies, obviously there is a much stronger likelihood the trigger is going to be pulled. If you take a multivitamin and put healthy, nutritious organic food in your body and maybe have a green drink (for which I'll give you the ingredients later in the book), obviously your genes are going to express completely differently. So, the environment determines the expression of your genes. And what that's called, instead of your genotype or your genotypic expression, is your phenotype, or your phenotypic expression.

When you start introducing these healthy lifestyle changes such as physical, chemical, and emotional/mental/spiritual changes, your genes express themselves in a healthier way, so you will always get healthier. Again, the level to which you can climb will be determined by how many physical limitations there are, what has been removed, how much damage has been done, how long you've been subluxated in your spine, and how long you've been taking any particular drug. The great news is that everybody can improve when they have interference removed, and the causes of their problems are addressed.

CHAPTER FOUR

THE NERVE SYSTEM: THE MASTER CONTROL SYSTEM

"Intellectuals solve problems; geniuses prevent them."
-Albert Einstein

When a sperm and an egg come together at conception, God breathes life into that cell, and within sixteen days, the first organ forms: the brain and central nervous system. Nothing forms before that central nervous system, not the heart, not the stomach; nothing shows up until you have a brain and a spinal cord. You can see this in photographs of embryonic development.

The central nervous system, comprising the brain, spinal cord, and spinal nerves, controls, coordinates, harmonizes, regulates, and governs every single aspect of health and healing and organ function from the cradle to the grave. Every single cell in your body is controlled, first and foremost, by this system. It's involved with every single function. It's involved in the digestion of food. It's involved in healing a cut on your hand. For your heart to beat and regulate properly, messages must travel from your brain through your spinal cord, along various nerves to your heart.

True health and healing comes from only one place. If you open up Gray's Anatomy, which is basically the bible for health-care students, it states that the central nervous system controls all function of the human body. So, if it controls all function, then we know that all health and healing comes from the brain.

There's a special branch of science called psychoneuroimmunology, which describes the connection between the brain, nerve system (central and peripheral), and the immune system. Scientists now know that your immune system is directly connected to the nervous system. Thoughts, feelings, emotions, and all the physical and chemical elements that we talked about earlier are tied in via the nervous system directly into the immune system.

Since we know that every organ and cell of the body are controlled through the nervous system and also that energy production is created on a cellular level, your nervous system, therefore, must control the energy production of the body.

A healthy lifestyle is critical for supporting real wellness, but is always secondary to a well functioning nervous system--the transmitter of life, healing, and function!

Energy flows from the brain through the spinal cord and the nerves, and out to every single organ. Messages travel in the form of electrical energy. If the nervous system is not working properly, that electrical energy will diminish, and therefore your body has less energy produced for it to use.

The nervous system regulates and runs off seventy millivolts of electrical potential. Neuro-scientists performed experiments many years ago with rabbits in which they hooked electrodes up to their brains and were able to power small light bulbs with the electrical potential generated. Like an electrical wire in your house or car, if a nerve is interrupted, there is no way for that energy to be moved. Whatever you are trying to power, whether a lamp, an organ, a muscle, or the healing of disease, will simply not occur if it does not get the energy it needs.

To be more specific about how energy is transported, there are seven cervical vertebrae (in the neck); twelve thoracic vertebrae (in the mid-back), and five lumbar vertebrae (in the lower back). You also have the sacrum and the coccyx at the bottom of your spine. These are the various parts of the spine. The most important part of the spine is the first bone in the neck, called the atlas vertebra. Of all 206 bones in the human anatomy, I feel that, clinically (and much of science concurs), the atlas vertebra is the most important bone of them all. It connects the brain to the spinal cord, and that connection in various cultures is referred to as the "mouth of God." Everything required for life and healing passes through that bone, and if it moves out of alignment, through emotional, physical, or chemical stress, it blocks life at the source. It's the area that Christopher Reeves injured, and the same one that my father injured. It sits all the way at the top of the neck and actually wraps around the brainstem area. Through it passes all the information that keeps us alive.

The neural components that pass through the atlas and the neural canal house 120 trillion nerve tracts that bring function to all parts of the body. If any of these bones move out of alignment, not just the atlas, there can be serious implications and health risks. This can occur due to falls, collisions, or injuries as an adult or a child. It can happen by lifting, turning, bending, or twisting improperly. It can be caused by the birth process (particularly with medical intervention); auto accidents; poor posture (computer work, long-distance driving, position at work, etc.); improper sitting and sleeping positions (including pillow and mattress problems); any physical, mental, or chemical stress (chemical stress is caused primarily by processed foods, medications, and environmental toxins); or lack of exercise, which can cause weak or tight muscles. Just as you can't keep driving a car without needing to tune it up, you can't use your body at 100% if it to is out of alignment. When bones move out of alignment creating neurological interference/disruption, this is known as vertebral subluxation. This is a serious condition: If any of the bones of the spine, particularly the top two bones of the spine (occiput and atlas) become slightly displaced, nerve tracts from the spinal cord can be impinged in varying degrees, interfering with the normal function of the body and preventing good health. The ultimate result is malfunction; serious limitation on health potential; eventual disease and potential death to the organs or areas lacking supply; and, of course, blockage of the full expression of human potential.

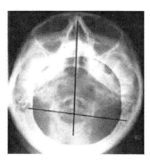

Really, if any of your vertebrae moves out of alignment, it can create neurological pressure or irritation to the spinal cord or its nerve filaments extending below. This causes short-circuiting to the nerve system, which causes aberrant nerve firing to the organs and most importantly up to the brain. That's when subluxation causes and contributes to sickness and disease. In other words, improper input equals improper output. This is supported by clinical observation and research and is the most devastating health condition one can find in the human body. It's worse than eating bad food; it's worse than not exercising; it's worse than thinking bad thoughts; it's worse than any of those things, because subluxation often has no obvious pain or symptoms and yet it destroys the system that runs your body. It's like having termites eating away at your house for years and years, and all of a sudden, one day, you walk across your kitchen floor and it collapses. You suddenly find yourself in your basement with a broken leg. That's what subluxation does neurologically. It slowly eats away without your body really knowing it and without sending you symptoms or pain signals. The reason for this is that at least 94 percent of the nervous system does not give you pain signals; only 6 percent of this system is designed to allow you to feel or is designated for sensory input.

There are many health conditions that may exist without overt signs or symptoms throughout their course, or without overt signs or symptoms until their end stages. Some of these include: arrhythmia, atherosclerosis, atrial fibrillation, atriventricular block, benign prostatic hypertrophy, breast cancer, Carcinoid syndrome, cardiomyopathy, cervix erosion, cervical spondylosis, cancer of the cervix, colorectal cancer, cholelithiasis, coccidioidomycosis, cor pulmonale, coronary artery disease, diabetes mellitus, diverticular disease, emphysema, encephalitis (viral or aseptic), fibroid tumors, glomerulonephritis, hyperbilirubinemia, hypertension, osteoarthritis, osteoporosis, ovarian cancer, ovarian cysts, Paget's disease, pilonidal cyst, polycystic kidney, polycythemia, polyps of large bowel, prostate cancer, pulmonary valve stenosis, pyelonephritis (chronic), renal calculi, renal failure (chronic), retinoblastoma, scoliosis, tooth decay, and tuberculosis.

People come to Yachter Family Chiropractic Center for many reasons: neck and back pain, heart disease, cancer, diabetes, infections, osteoporosis, high blood pressure, high cholesterol, hyperactivity, learning disorders, asthma, allergies, Parkinson's, Alzheimer's, multiple sclerosis, fibromyalgia, chronic fatigue, intestinal disease, aches and pains, and paralysis, and many health conditions too numerous to name.

Chiropractors do not heal these specific conditions or diseases. We aim to maximize the function of the nervous system, which in turn will allow the body full God-given healing potential and full-human performance. This principle has stood the test of time and helped millions of people world-wide for over a century.

RESEARCH ON THE SPINE, THE ATLAS, AND SUBLUXATION

- As described earlier, atlas subluxations affect organ function. This has been demonstrated in the gastrointestinal tract, urinary bladder, adrenal medulla, lymphatic tissues, heart, vessels of the brain, and peripheral nerves (Journal of Manipulative Physiol Therapeutics Nov-Dec; 18 (9): 597-602 1995).

- Burl Pettibon, founder of The Pettibon System of Spinal Correction), found in 2005, that 98.7% of children with ADD have subluxated atlas bones."

- A study published in the Journal of the American Osteopathic Association found that out of 1,250 infants chosen at random, 211 suffered from nervousness, vomiting, muscular abnormalities, tremors and insomnia. Two hundred of those children had abnormal cervical (neck) muscle strain indicating vertebral subluxation. When the subluxation was adjusted and the muscle strain removed, an immediate calming often resulted; the children's crying stopped, the muscles relaxed, and the children fell asleep. The authors noted that an unhealthy spine causes "many clinical features from central motor impairment to lower resistance to infections – especially ear, nose, and throat infections."

- Decreased blood flow from abnormal posture is a major factor in all disease, including cancer. Reich W. *The Discovery of the Orgone*. New York; The Noonday Press, 197.

- THE SEALY INSTITUTE HAS FOUND THAT POSTURE AFFECTS AND MODERATES EVERY PHYSICAL FUNCTION OF THE BODY: The Sealy Institute has made observations of the striking influence posture mechanics has on function and symptomatology that has led to their hypothesis that posture effects and moderates every physiologic function from breathing to hormonal production. Spinal pain, blood pressure, headaches, pulse, lung capacity and mood are only a small portion of the body's functions that are most easily influenced by posture. The most significant influences of posture are upon respiration, oxygenation, and nerve function. Ultimately, it appears that homeostasis (balance) and autonomic regulation are intimately connected with posture. The corollary of these observations is that many symptoms, including pain, may be moderated or eliminated by improving posture. J Lennon,

BM, MM, C N Sealy, MD, R K Cady, MD, W Matta, PhD, R Cox, PhD, and W F Simpson, PhD, "Postural and Respiratory Modulation of Autonomic Function, Pain and Health". AJPM Vol. 4 No.1 January 1994 pp 36-39.

- Dr. J. Freeman found over 50 years ago that shifts in the body's center of gravity due to aging cause postural deviations leading to intestinal diverticula, hemorrhoids, varicosities of the legs, osteoporosis, hip and foot deformities, overall poor health and quality of life, as well as, even shortened life span. Freeman JT. "Posture In The Aging And Aged Body". JAMA 1957;165 (7): pp843-846.

- Dr. Rene Cailliet, Director of the Department of Physical Medicine and Rehabilitation, University of Southern California, reached the following conclusions regarding the mechanical derangement of both hard and soft tissues of the spine and the patients' posture. They are:

1. Lordotic curves of the cervical and lumbar spine are necessary for normal spinal function.

2. With a forward-extended head posture, normal lordosis is lost in both the cervical and lumbar spine, which in turn mechanically blocks optimal spinal function.

3. Head forward posture can add up to thirty (30) pounds of abnormal leverage on the spine; therefore, abnormal position of the head can pull the entire spine out of alignment.

4. Forward head posture results in loss of vital capacity. Lung capacity is depleted by as much as 30%. Shortness of breath can then lead to heart and blood vascular disease.

5. The entire gastrointestinal system is affected; particularly the large intestine. Loss of good bowel parastolic function and evacuation are a common sequel to forward head posture with loss of spinal curvatures.

6. Forward head posture with loss of cervical lordosis causes an increase in discomfort and pain. Motions of the first four cervical vertebrae are blocked. Normal movement of these vertebrae is a necessary stimulus for endorphin production by the brain and spinal cord. With inadequate endorphin production, many otherwise non-painful sensations are experienced as pain.

7. Forward head position altars head-spine posture and stance, as well as ones gait and body motions. One becomes hunched. The entire body becomes rigid and all body motions are lessened. The better the posture, the better one looks and feels.

Cailliet R, M.D., Gross L, Rejuvenation Strategy. New York, Doubleday Co. 1987.

- Dr. Alf Alfred Breig, neurosurgeon and Nobel Prize recipient discovered that a loss of the cervical curve can stretch the spinal cord 5 to 7 cm and produce pathological tension, putting the body in a state of disease." –Alfred Breig, neurosurgeon and Nobel Prize recipient.

- Every inch of forward head posture, it can increase the weight of the head on the spine by an additional 10 pounds." (Kapandji, Physiology of The Joints, Vol. 3).

WHAT POSTURAL/SPINAL RESEARCH HAS CONCLUDED IS:

1. Posture affects all human functions, both consciously and unconsciously, from breathing to thinking.

2. Posture affects breathing and vital capacity, as well as influences vocal sounds. If sound is not optimally vocalized, the individual does not experience vocal expression.

3. Posture reflects mind and body interaction. Inefficient posture and resultant poor breathing eventually leads to pathologic dysfunction.

4. People with good posture ventilate and oxygenate their bodies optimally. These people sit and stand straight and tall. They invariably exude vitality and project a commanding vocal presence. That elusive attribute referred to as charisma appears to be a state of mind reflected in the visual and audible presence of individuals with properly adjusted posture.

5. Correct spinal position and correct posture allow physical activities that improve mental and physical health and feelings of well being. Feeling of mental and physical well being appears to encourage the person to further exude confidence that is reflected in their posture, stance and gait.

Spinal damage can happen if you're tense or under a lot of stress. Stress causes the release of hormones such as cortisol and adrenaline that tighten the muscles around the spine. Those tight muscles can pull and shift the bones out of alignment, causing degeneration, which in turn causes bones to pinch into the spinal cord and push and compress the spinal nerve. Stress can also come from chemicals. For instance, if you put a lot of white sugar into your body, the white toxic poison, you can cause loss of muscle tone. When that happens, the bones can shift out of alignment and press into the spinal cord, causing more electrical misfiring and more problems.

You can take many steps to protect the spine. I would start with sleeping posture. Also, when you're working at a computer or sitting all day, make sure you have the right posture. If you're lifting, turning, bending or twisting, know how to position your body properly. If you're doing athletics, warm up with the proper exercises. Weight-lifters need to learn techniques that protect the spine and its curves.

In our office, chiropractic adjustments are given primarily to structurely restore proper spinal alignment. We also prescribe special spinal exercises that help restore the normal curvatures in the spine, thereby relaxing the spinal cord. The spine has three curves, but the most important one is in the neck. In our clinic, we call it the Arc of Life. Published scientific research has shown that the ideal is a 43- to 45-degree arc in the neck. This is because when the neck is curved, the spinal cord is relaxed or slackened, allowing maximum neurological delivery of impulses out to your body. We have specific exercises designed to induce the cervical curve back into your neck. There are stretches and exercises that train muscle memory to naturally induce a lordosis (curve) into the neck. We also have neck traction, wobble board exercises, and whole-body vibration technology at Yachter Family Chiropractic Center (YFCC) to assist in spinal correction.

HERE IS THE PURPOSE AND BENEFIT OF EACH IN-OFFICE SPINAL CORRECTIVE EXERCISE AT YACHTER FAMILY CHIROPRACTIC (YFCC):

1. Wobble Chair and Neck Traction:

   - Adds strength and flexibility to the discs and ligaments of the low back.

- Reduces stress in the low back and aids in the prevention and recuperation of injuries.

- Assists in the healing of torn and/or bulging discs.

- Rehydrates/inflates the lumbar discs and keeps them young, strong and healthy.

- Helps circulate cerebro-spinal fluid CSF (fluid that nourishes the brain and spinal cord). By providing regular stimulation and nourishment for the brain, this can possibly stave off neurodegenerative diseases like Alzheimer's and Parkinson's disease.

- Massages heart (via central tendon) and reduces the chance of a heart attack.

- Stimulates reflexes to correct posture (when wearing body weights).

- Enhances oxygenation of blood and stimulates metabolism, which is necessary for the prevention of disease.

- Warms up the discs prior to the adjustment and prior to spinal molding at home to reshape the spine more easily.

2. Head/shoulder/hip weights:

- Corrects forward head posture and overall posture.

- Relieves tension on the spinal cord, helping energy to flow easier from the brain into the body and restoring overall health.

- Relieves stress/tension on the heart.

- Promotes tissue oxygenation by increasing lung capacity.

- Relieves pressure and stress on degenerative discs and damaged ligaments so they can rehydrate/regenerate and heal.

- Strengthens weakened neck muscles.

- When worn immediately after the adjustment or at home after cervical traction/wobble chair, the body-weighting system helps hold and stabilize spinal corrections longer to accelerate results.

3. Vibe Plate (whole body vibration):

- Increases muscle strength, tone, and endurance.

- Helps correct the loss of cervical curve.

- Improves posture, coordination, and balance.

- Increases growth hormone and increases anti-aging hormone by up to 361 percent.

- Increases testosterone, libido, and energy.

- Increases immune function.

- Decreases pain and inflammation.

- Accelerates weight loss, and helps reduce appearance of cellulite

- Improves deep intrinsic spinal muscle responses promoting spinal stability, essential for individuals suffering from pain due to surgery and chronic spinal instability.

- Aids in detoxification and removal of wastes from the body.

- Improves function and thereby improves health. Increases bone density (by 34 percent over one year), which helps decrease development of osteoporosis..

- Helps reduce arthritic pain, joint, and ligament stress

- Enhances critical blood flow in the body (oxygenation and lymph drainage).

- Helps relieve menopausal symptoms.

- Increases serotonin (the "happiness" hormone).

- Improves neurocognition and neuroadaptation – extremely important for patients with neurodegenerative disease (Alzheimer's/Parkinson's/multiple sclerosis) and traumatic injury.

- Enhances explosive strength and fast twitch muscles and speeds training recovery

A MAP OF MISALIGNMENT

An X-ray can show the position of the subluxation. Then, to locate interference or neurological distortion, we use thermography and EMG (electromyography, which records the electrical activity of muscles). In addition to the spinal X-rays and examination of posture, technological advances have brought forth tests such as the EMG as well as computerized range-of-motion and muscle evaluations. These provide even more insight into the presence of neurological interference, abnormal spinal alignment, mal-position of the spinal curves, joint degeneration, and other parts of the vertebral subluxation complex.

In general, the EMG is primarily concerned with how neurons are firing into muscles. Thermal values, generated from the thermography technology can be used as a standard in assessment of sympathetic nerve function, and the degree of asymmetry (measured via standard deviation) is a quantifiable indicator of dysfunction/ improper nerve function. These tools measure what X-rays can't. Because these diagnosing practices are so multifaceted, together they provide a complete picture of the patient's spinal and overall health.

On the next page is a picture of a thermal scan reading obtained in our clinic using the CLA Insight Millenium Technology, invented by Dr. Chris Kent and Dr. Patrick Gentempo. White, dark gray, and gray would indicate less intense neurological distortion, while black would indicate more severe.

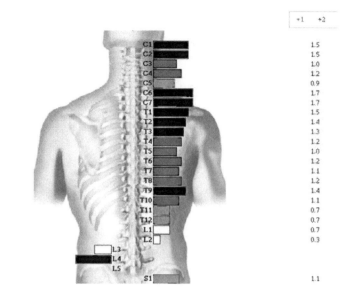

Scientists have found that posture affects and moderates every physical and mental function in the body. Spinal pain, blood pressure, headaches, pulse, lung capacity, and mood are only a small portion of the body's functions that are most easily influenced by posture.

—Dr. C. Norman Shealy, Shealy Institute

It's never too late and never too early to have your neurological system evaluated. I check babies at birth. My brother, also a chiropractor, checked his children as they were being delivered. Usually hours after a birth I'm evaluating the nervous system, doing scans and palpation. Babies' bones are not totally ossified in all places, so when I check them it's very different from an adult adjustment. It's a soft, vibrational stimulus on the neck or spine, and the bone moves because of the vibrational force that's introduced.

THE FIRST SUBLUXATION

Dr. Gotfried Guttman, M.D., once staff member of the Department of Pathology, Boston University School of Medicine, Mallory Institute of Pathology, found that childhood subluxations had received "far too little attention." Because of the frequency of problems, especially at birth, he recommended a chiropractic spinal checkup as soon as possible after delivery. "Mechanical injury to the upper cervical spinal structures is indicated as a causal mechanism in cases of Sudden Infant Death Syndrome."

Every adult, every child, every human being on the planet should have his or her spine evaluated from the beginning of life, since clinically we now know that it is the most critical element of being healthy.

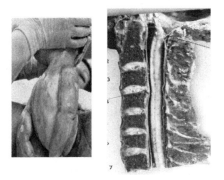

CHIROPRACTIC AND DEGENERATIVE

NEUROLOGICAL DISORDERS

Spinal correction and lifestyle direction for degenerative neurological disorders such as multiple sclerosis and Parkinson's can result in tremendous benefits. Multiple sclerosis is a gradual breaking down of the spinal cord. What we have found clinically is M.S. patients benefit enormously from a healthy nerve system. There are several patients at our office who are now in complete remission from the symptoms of this awful disease.

A study evaluating the care of forty-four MS patients and thirty-seven Parkinson's patients who received treatment of upper neck subluxation (atlas) over a five-year period revealed that 91 percent of MS patients showed improvement and 92 percent of Parkinson's patients showed improvement. These findings led researchers to believe that the adjustment of spinal subluxations in the upper cervical spine could activate a reversal of MS and Parkinson's symptoms. For a long time, head and neck injuries have been thought of as contributing factors to the development of MS and Parkinson's. These results are the first to confirm the relationship between the two.

CHIROPRACTIC CUTS BLOOD PRESSURE

Study Finds Special "Atlas Adjustment" Lowers Blood Pressure

A recent placebo-controlled study suggests chiropractic adjustment can significantly lower high blood pressure. According to the study leader, Dr. George Bakris, director of the University of Chicago hypertension center, chiropractic adjustments have the effect of not one, but two blood pressure medications given in combination. The study showed that there were no side-effects.

Eight weeks after undergoing the procedure, 25 patients with early-stage high blood pressure had significantly lower blood pressure than 25 similar patients who underwent a sham chiropractic adjustment. Because patients couldn't feel the technique, they were unable to tell which group they were in. X-rays showed that the procedure realigned the atlas vertebra – the doughnut-like bone at the very top of the spine – with the spine in the treated patients, but not in the sham-treated patients. Compared to the sham-treated patients, those who got the real procedure saw an average 14 mm Hg greater drop in systolic blood pressure (the top number in a blood pressure count), and an average 8 mm Hg greater drop in diastolic blood pressure (the bottom blood pressure number).

None of the patients took blood pressure medicine during the eight-week study.

CHIROPRACTIC AND THE IMMUNE SYSTEM

There is a powerful connection between the spine, nerve system, and the immune system. The following are several studies that prove the powerful affect of chiropractic adjustments on the overall performance of the immune system:

- Canadian Memorial University conducted a study of Interleukin II, which has long been known to stimulate T-lymphocytes to fight cancer growth and viral and bacterial infections. Researchers found that after one thoracic (mid-back) chiropractic adjustment, Interleukin II was immediately elevated for a period of two hours. Kyron pharmaceutical company produces synthetic Interleukin ("Proleukin") for treatment of renal cell carcinoma, malignant melanoma, and viral infections, and it is used as an immune system booster vaccine for AIDS treatment. Each Proleukin treatment ranges from several thousand to tens of thousands of dollars.

- Dr. Ronald Pero found at the New York University Cancer Prevention Research Center that chiropractic patients under regular wellness care for five years or more had immune systems that were on the average 200 percent stronger than those patients not under chiropractic care.

PREGNANCY AND CHIROPRACTIC

Startling new research shows a possible link between spinal adjustments and increased fertility in some women. "It lets couples who have been infertile or couples who are planning on having a family [have] hope," explains Dr. Madeline Behrendt. She led a study of fifteen women who struggled with infertility, some for more than a decade. Each went to see Dr. Behrendt for a variety of problems, not for infertility. Of the fifteen women, fourteen became pregnant. "The chiropractor identifies spinal distortions, which are called subluxations, and once they were detected and corrected, the fertility function improved," Dr. Behrendt explains. She says there's a link between chiropractic care and fertility because the nerves to your reproductive system run through your spine. She says that when the back is misaligned, the nerves misfire and cause a hormone imbalance, which can prevent a woman from getting pregnant. Dr. Behrendt is now on a mission to see more research dollars spent on the benefits of chiropractic care and infertility.

Chiropractic is also important for expectant mothers. Nerve impulses into the womb will play an integral role in the child's progress. Structurally, the child is at rest inside the pelvic cavity. Spinal distortion, pelvic rotation, and subluxation can all have a negative effect on not only the likelihood of conception but also on development and delivery. In studies conducted within the medical profession, it was shown that women who received chiropractic adjustments in their third trimester of pregnancy were able to carry and deliver children with more comfort and that those incorporating chiropractic adjustments during their pregnancy needed half as much painkiller during delivery.

THE SUPREMACY OF THE NERVOUS SYSTEM

Exercise is an integral part of health. However, exercising in the presence of subluxation is not as beneficial. A physical therapist can exercise the muscles of someone who is paralyzed; however, the therapist's efforts do not help those muscle fibers that have no nerve supply. The exercise will only benefit the muscles where the damage to the nerve system has not occurred and there is good electrical communication. You can exercise muscles regularly, but if they are not receiving a full supply of life from the nervous system, they will be deprived of proper nutrition and growth.

A good diet is extremely important. The body can't live on caffeine and doughnuts alone. It needs good nutrition to make healthy organs and tissues. But nutritious food cannot build living, healthy tissue unless it has electrical life coming from the brain to convert it into usable material to support the body. If life and the healing force are lacking in the body due to subluxation, the body will not be able to assimilate or absorb the full nutrient value form that food.

Rest is important to rebuild tissues and the body in general. But unless the body is receiving proper nerve supply, it will be deprived of adequate rest. Everyone has had the experience of waking up tired and groggy even after a full night's sleep. The chemical changes that must take place within the body while sleeping will go awry if the glands, organs, and various systems of the body do not have good nerve communication. Subluxation steals your body's ability to regenerate and rejuvenate itself.

CHAPTER FIVE

PROFILE OF A
BALANCED BODY

"Energy and persistence conquer all things."
-Benjamin Franklin

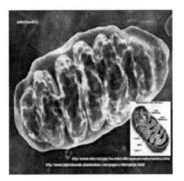

(Mitochondria: energy production factory of the human cell)

Energy is a representation of your true level of health. People who are healthier have a higher level of energy, and those who are sicker have less energy. Human cells generate enormous amounts of energy. Sick, diseased, cells don't. Energy management means doing things that will protect your energy level, maximize your energy production, and thus keep you in the best of health; this will allow you to achieve everything that you were created to achieve and contribute the most to those around you.

We get more energy by fueling our bodies properly, directing our thoughts properly, and moving our bodies properly. To do that, we must put the right things into our bodies and our minds, and pay attention to those three primary areas of interference: physical, emotional, and chemical. As interference is lessened, the natural energy of the body will be expressed.

LET'S LOOK AT THE THREE
SOURCES OF ENERGY:

Putting the right foods in your body is top priority. The foods that add the highest quality resources to energize the body are chemical-free, plant-based, and organic. That means lots of vegetables, some fruits, whole, unprocessed grains (preferably sprouted); nuts and seeds (preferably water soaked), and legumes. If you choose to eat dairy and meat, you want it chemical-free, nonpasteurized, and organic; such as meat that has been grass-fed and not grain-fed (the omega-6 fats in grain-fed meats have an inflammatory and energy-draining effect on the human body).

You also want to eat foods low in sugar because in the long term, sugar destroys energy; it does not create it. I once heard a pastor call it "white death." Avoid trans-fats at all costs, choosing instead good mono- and polyunsaturated fats found in avocados, olive oil, flaxseed oil, fish oils, almonds, and walnuts; these are healthy fats that help create energy and give your cells the building blocks and the resources to generate an enormous amount of energy.

The second source of energy comes from moving your body. Every human being should move around at least thirty minutes a day, every day. When you go to the mall, don't park in the closest spot. Park at the perimeter and walk. Movement creates energy. It gets your spine moving, thus your nervous system working, and oxygen pumping; it gets the lymphatic system flowing through your body, which eliminates wastes and toxins. The lymphatic system is like the gutter of your body. It collects all the refuse and toxins, junk and acids; but if you don't move, that stuff doesn't get pushed out and moved out of your body. The pump for your lymphatic system is not your heart, it's your muscles.

The third source of energy comes from thinking the right thoughts and avoiding the toxic mindsets that cripple us emotionally and spiritually. Many studies have shown that being positive, enthusiastic, and encouraging makes us feel better in general. We have more energy and better mental clarity when we are around positive people speaking positive words. And try to notice next time that you're around a negative person; watch how fast you start to have negative thoughts: It drains you, it decreases your energy. These are some of the things we need to think about if we are to create tremendous energy and manage it properly. We want to create more energy so we can do the things we love to do in life. Energy makes it possible to accomplish our dreams and goals. It allows us to complete our mission in life. It lets us contribute more, grow more, give more, serve more, love more, and become all that God has created us to be. It allows us to serve our brothers and sisters and to leave a positive, loving legacy for generations, as God would have us do.

So why do we want more energy? To be a better parent and spouse, to be a better teacher or CEO, to be a better doctor, lawyer, minister, accountant, or whatever it is you do in life that makes a positive impact; it all requires energy.

YOU CONTROL FOOD OR IT CONTROLS YOU
AND YOUR ENERGY LEVEL
ALKALINE BY DESIGN

The intracellular fluids of the body should be maintained at a 7.365 pH level. Our body is created to be alkaline by design, but acidic by function. The metabolic functions produce acid, but just like a battery, you want your pH balance to be alkaline because an alkaline environment provides the highest level of electrochemical potential. And also just like a battery, our bodies work off of electrochemical potential.

To be more specific, our nervous system works off of seventy millivolts of electrical potential; the kidneys and liver work off of forty millivolts. Certain foods will either fuel the system by adding alkalinity, or take away energy by adding acidity. All in all, the body maintains an optimal level of health and well-being when it stays slightly alkaline. That is the goal for biochemical balance with less interference and high energy production.

Acidity can be measured in potential hydrogen (pH). We can think of this as the power of hydrogen, the simplest element -- a single proton and electron. The pH measures the electrical potential, or the amount of protons and electrons, in a food or substance. The more electron-rich a food is, the more alkaline it's going to be. The more proton-rich a food is, the more acidic it's going to be. We want our food selections to be at least 70 to 80 percent alkaline or electron-rich. When electrons go into the body, they increase electrical or energy potential. The safe and effective way to have health, energy, and vitality is to simply maintain the alkaline design of the body with an alkaline lifestyle and diet.

ACID EROSION AND DAMAGE

Acidic blood wreaks havoc on many systems of the body, including the blood vessels. Acidic blood causes abrasions and irritations to the blood vessel walls, resulting in a sheering force. The rush of acidic blood through the arteries peals the artery lining off and can throw off an embolus. Cholesterol then comes to the rescue to repair the wall and cover the abrasive tear. The cholesterol helps make the area waterproof to repair the tear. This repairing cholesterol, low-density lipoprotein (LDL) is a life saver, not an artery clogger. This type of cholesterol is usually called bad cholesterol, but it is simply doing its job to save you. The fastest way to save a person from clogged arteries is to increase alkaline food selections and increase intake of good clean, alkaline water (more about that later); all of this will contribute to diluting the deleterious effects of the acidic bloodstream. Cholesterol drugs are highly injurious: They do not get to the cause of high cholesterol levels and cause significant side-effect damage. These drugs have been linked to cancer, heart disease, memory loss, severe joint and muscle pain, and even sudden heart attack.

"When man violates man's laws, we send him to jail and point the finger of scorn at him. When he violates nature's laws, we send him to a hospital, give him flowers, and feel sorry for him."

B. J. Palmer, developer of chiropractic

The longest nerve in the body, the vagus, which runs from the brain to the lower body, deteriorates from acidic exposure due to dietary and metabolic acids. The vagus nerve is the main neural component of the parasympathetic nervous system, or that part of the nervous system that takes care of functions that run more or less on autopilot. These include heart rate, immune system function, respiratory function, a man's ability to have an erection, and digestion. As we age, the vagus nerve is affected and damaged by rising blood acid levels. These affects can be measured in increases in heart rate, the increase in erectile impotence in men, and digestive problems.

GREEN-PLANT FOODS ARE IDEAL
FOR ENERGY PRODUCTION

Blood is liquid tissue. It's the river of life, as microbiologist and best-selling author Dr. Robert O. Young refers to it. We must keep it clean and flowing, and green-plant foods are the ideal way to do this. Green foods are some of the lowest-calorie, low-sugar, and nutrient-rich foods on the planet. The green color is produced by chlorophyll, the "blood" of the plants. Its molecular structure is similar to the hemoglobin of human blood. Hemoglobin is the body's oxygen transporter. The components of chlorophyll are almost identical to those of hemoglobin. A German chemist, Dr. Richard Wohlstetter, determined in 1913 that the two molecules closely resemble one another. He found that hemoglobin is composed of four elements: carbon, hydrogen, oxygen, and nitrogen. Hemoglobin to iron content is the main reason we need a dietary supply of that mineral. Chlorophyll has the same elements; however, they are organized around a single atom of magnesium, not iron. Chlorophyll reduces the binding of carcinogens (cancer-causing agents) to DNA, the liver, and other organs. It also breaks down calcium oxalate stones, which are created by the body to neutralize and dispose of excess acid. The best sources of chlorophyll are wheat grass and barley grass. As Dr. Young states in his writings, "Grass, this little plant we walk on and usually take for granted, is a doorway to health." Grass has the power to regenerate our bodies at the molecular and cellular level and help us significantly increase our energy level.

There is a balance in nature as well as in the bloodstream, and one example of the expression of this balance is the tightly linked biochemistry of the two essential fatty acid groups, the omega-6 and omega-3 oils. Unlike other fats, neither is made in the human body; rather, these essential fatty acids are synthesized in the chloroplasts of plants. The chloroplasts, the green chlorophyll-containing structure of plant cells, convert sunlight and carbon dioxide into oxygen and a range of complex organic molecules, including: sugars, proteins, and fats. Only chloroplasts within certain plants (i.e., marine and fresh-water algae) produce high quantities of long-chain omega-3 fatty acids. Fish feed upon this algae, which is why fish are a great source of fat and nutrition for the whole body and brain.

According to Dr. Bircher-Benner, a visionary pioneer in holistic, natural healing, "Absorption and organization of sunlight, the very essence of life, is almost exclusively derived from plants. Plants are therefore a biological accumulation of light. Since light is the driving force of every cell in our bodies, that is why we need plants."

BUILDING A NEW HOUSE

There is a new paradigm called the House of Health. It's a new way of eating, as opposed to the old food triangle or food squares that we used to follow in school. Those models are distorted and inaccurate and actually made a lot of people sick and tired. The foundation of that triangle is a lot of refined and processed starchy carbohydrates such as breads, pastas, cereals and grains that pour tons of sugar into your body and make you rapidly gain lots of fat. By increasing your blood sugar, you increase your insulin levels. This leads to an increased chance of obesity and diabetes along with a weakened immune system. This is partly why we're the most obese country in the world.

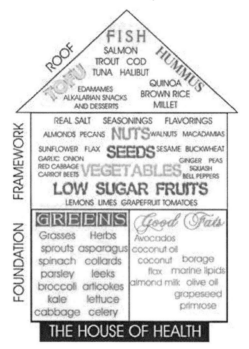

The House of Health was developed by Dr. Young, Ph.D., D.Sc., and his wife, Shelley Redford Young, LMT. It suggests that 60 to 80 percent of food selections should be alkaline. It's based on a foundation of lots of green foods and good fats making up at least 50 to 60 percent of the recommended diet; other alkaline choices that bring the level up to 70 or 80 percent are tomatoes, grapefruits, lemons, and limes, and other highly alkalizing fruits, as well as edamame (whole soy) beans, and grains like spelt. These foods will naturally detoxify your body, pulling out acidity, resulting in increasing energy. Higher energy is a natural expression of an alkaline body, and that's what the House of Health will do for you.

One of my most often-quoted statements is: "When the fish is sick, change the water." We don't feed fish medicine. We need clean water. When the cells of our body are sick, we must change the water and fluids in which all cells and tissues are bathed.

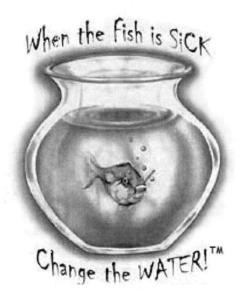

"The soul must see through these eyes alone, and if they are dim, the whole world is clouded."

— *Johann Wolfgang von Goethe*

DISEASE AND TOXICITY:

GENETICS OR LIFESTYLE?

The two causes of disease are toxicity and deficiency. Dr. Young's New Biology tells us that alkalizing the body will help to maximize your body's detoxification processes as well as replenish deficient vitamins, minerals, antioxidants, phytonutrients, good fats, proteins, carbohydrates, and hydration.

According to the University of Columbia School of Public Health, "Ninety-five percent of all cancer and disease are due to diet and the accumulation of toxins." Depending upon the source, the numbers range from 60 to 97 percent. If this is true, then our chance of developing cancer lies within our control and is heavily determined by our lifestyle choices.

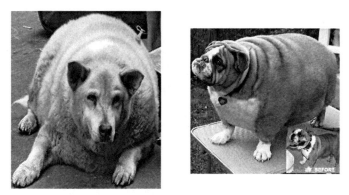

GENETICS OR LIFESTYLE?

Do the pictures above show animals with thyroid conditions, diabetes, bad genetics, glandular problems, bad luck, or just bad lifestyle? When you see these animals, what comes to mind first? Do you wonder how they got that way – genetics or lifestyle? Perhaps your comment would be: "Stop feeding the animal so much junk!" I think we'd all agree that to a large degree we create disease with our mouths;

we don't just wake up and catch disease. Again, unless we have had our body physically altered (i.e., organs removed), we have the power to alter our health to a large degree.

Think about it this way: Would you get up in the morning and give your dog or cat a cup of coffee, a cigarette, and a doughnut? Or pour sand into the gas tank of your car? Many of us don't realize the human body needs proper fuel to run efficiently and energize the body's approximately 200 trillion cells. Diseases that are almost entirely caused by "lifestyle choices" include obesity, degenerative disease, retention of water, plaque formation, depression, diabetes, inflammatory conditions, high triglycerides, high cholesterol, cancer, skin disorders, osteoporosis, and wrinkles. (Here's an energy enhancing tip: No late-night snacking. The digestive process while you sleep robs you of vital healing energy and an energy drain the next day.)

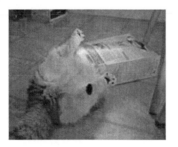

GET YOUR HYDRATION!

The body is up to 60 percent water, and just through day-to-day perspiration and urination we lose incredible amounts of fluid. To properly flush out the toxins, we need to be fully hydrated, and that takes a lot of water. Every cell in the body is a toxic, acid-manufacturing plant. Cells produce energy, but at the same time release acid, toxins, and carbon dioxide; sort of the way a car's tailpipe emits carbon monoxide. This is the stuff we need to flush out on a regular basis.

If you're working in an office space, you need to get up at least once per hour and flush these toxins out of your body. Drinking half your body weight in ounces is ideal. If you're trying to detoxify and are really in an energy slump, or if you're trying to heal from a disease, you want to actually make that one quart per every thirty pounds of body weight, and you'd want to do that for at least two to four weeks. It's a lot of water, but many people who are reading this book need to literally superhydrate their bodies if they're going to elevate their level of health and energy and do it quickly.

Some sources are better than others. The best water is alkalized and ionized. Ionization means that the water is made electron-rich, adding electrons to your body. It has enormous health benefits. I just got back from Alaska not too long ago, and I was able to bend down while walking on a glacier and drink 'virgin' glacier water. It's highly ionized and alkalized, and it was the best-tasting water I've ever had. When I drank it, it made my entire body tingle. It was like drinking a powerful drug. If you don't want to relocate, machines that do this are easy to find and range in price from $1,200 to $4,000. Reverse osmosis is the number two choice for drinking water, and after that would be distilled. Distilled water is completely pure, but it is devoid of minerals, and if you don't add minerals with something like a green drink, it will actually leach minerals out of your body.

God designed fruits and vegetables to contain naturally distilled water, so if you eat a lot of healthy, fresh foods, you won't have to drink as much water. Then, of course, your typical bottled water would probably be the least desirable choice. Bottled water, at least in plastic bottles, isn't recommended on a daily basis because pthalates are released from the plastic, which can toxify your brain and body. Pthalates can throw off the body's chemical-hormonal balance and possibly cause cancer. Pthalates are estrogen-like molecules found in a variety of chemical compounds such as household cleaning agents, paints, consumer products such as shampoo, soap, makeup, and plastic bottles. These pthalates fill estrogen receptor sites in the body and contribute to a condition called estrogen dominance, which can primarily lead to uterine and breast cancer. I drink out of glass as much as I can, even though it can be inconvenient or even hazardous to carry around. There are also stainless-steel canteens, which would be the next best selection, but even that material has the tendency to leach.

Unfortunately, the body's dehydration alert mechanisms are not very efficient. And as we age, they get less effective. By the time we have dry lips or dry skin and by the time we feel lethargic, we're extraordinarily dehydrated. The typical signs of dehydration are actually delayed, giving us an inaccurate picture of how hydrated our bodies are. Lack of water is the number-one trigger of daytime fatigue. Without enough water, you won't have energy. You'll feel tired and weak. A mere 2 percent drop in body water can trigger fuzzy short-term memory, trouble with basic math, and difficulty focusing on the computer screen or printed page. Even mild dehydration will slow down one's metabolism as much as 3 percent.

As a rule, you should be sipping every five to fifteen minutes. You should be taking mouthfuls of water throughout the day; this is the easiest way to drink about half your body weight in ounces each day. Don't wait until you have signs of dehydration; just get the water into your body. Water is the conduit of all life and the most essential nutrient to every metabolic function. According to the world's foremost authority on human hydration and internationally renowned researcher, Dr. Fereydoon Batmanghelidj, M.D., 90 percent of society is currently dehydrated, with 70 percent suffering unknowingly from dehydration-induced symptoms on a regular basis. Aching joints can be a sign of dehydration, which results in over-acidity. Dehydration predisposes a person to DNA damage, reduced efficiency of DNA repair, and immune system suppression which can lead to a much greater likelihood of cancer growth. Cancer cells love a dehydrated/ acidic environment because they thrive in low-oxygen, anaerobic/ acidic environments.

Additional complications of dehydration, according to Dr. Batmanghelidj, are as follows:

- EARLY MORNING SICKNESS
- HEARTBURN
- MIGRAINE HEADACHE
- ANGINA (CHEST AND ARM PAIN)
- RHEUMATOID JOINT PAIN
- BACK PAIN
- FIBROMYALGIA
- LEG PAIN
- COLITIS PAIN
- OBESITY
- RAISED CHOLESTEROL
- CHRONIC FATIGUE
- MULTIPLE SCLEROSIS
- PROSTATE/URINATION PROBLEMS
- OSTEOPOROSIS AND OSTEOARTHRITIS
- ALZHEIMER'S DISEASE

- STROKES

- INSULIN-DEPENDENT DIABETES

- AUTO-IMMUNE DISEASES

Your muscles, ligaments, discs, joints, and nerves constantly need hydration. I instruct all my patients that hydration is critical to maintaining a healthy spine and nerve system. Hydration is vital for the spine in so many ways:

1. It detoxifies waste materials from the discs.

2. Your nervous system uses water to carry neurotransmitters or messages from your brain along the nerves to all your organs and tissues.

3. Water cushions shock by surrounding the vertebral discs and joint cartilage.

4. The nervous system needs water and electrolytes (sea salt) to communicate properly.

THE HUMAN BODY WAS NOT DESIGNED TO FALL APART

Nobel Prize winner Dr. Alexis Carrel was able to keep cells from a chicken heart alive and replicating new cells for twenty-eight years, far outliving the life span of a chicken, which is seven to twelve years. The cells did not die of aging; the researchers simply terminated the experiment. Carroll writes, "The cell is immortal. It is merely the fluid in which it floats that degenerates. Renew this fluid at regular intervals, give the cell what it requires for nutrition, and as far as we know, the pulsation of life can go on forever."

THE PRISTINE SALT

Along those lines, sea salt is a vital detoxifying and balancing agent. It hasn't changed for eons, which means no contamination—that can't be said for other types of salt. For example, certain fields in Utah have been covered to protect them from environmental and soil toxins, and the salt in them contains, in most situations, the many minerals inherent in natural sea salt, without the contaminants. If you scooped seawater out of the sea and evaporated the water, the leftover salt contains all the vital life mineral elements that are supposed to be found together, intact, the way God created them. Sea salt contains all the minerals your body needs: calcium, copper, magnesium, manganese, phosphorus, potassium, and iron. They're all there, along with many, many others. Your body needs a daily supply and a full complement of these minerals.

Iodine also occurs naturally in sea salt, and we know that when people don't get iodine, their thyroid malfunctions. So it's critical that we take these minerals together in the form of sea salt so our bodies can regulate properly. Without a full supply of minerals, the organs of our body cannot be healthy; they cannot regulate properly, and they will develop disease.

In a 1997 article in the *American Journal of Clinical Nutrition*, Dr. David McCurran stated that with adequate daily intake of sea salt, which contains all vital elemental minerals [mainly magnesium for proper heart regulation], we have salt that will not raise blood pressure; but in fact, may actually lower it.

Sea salt helps the body detoxify on a cellular level. Every organ in the body requires salt to run properly because it relates to electrical potential. Vital life-giving communication is sent from the brain to the body through the nervous system. The heart and skeletal muscles require magnesium, which gives you an idea how important this element is. I drink a quarter teaspoon of sea salt in a quart of water every morning for deep cellular detoxification. The sea salt helps push lots of water into my cells quickly, at the same time pushing the toxic, acidic residue out. The sea salt aids in the normal functioning of the cellular pump known as the sodium/potassium pump, which again is indirectly responsible for bringing nourishment into the cell and expelling waste out of the cell. As that residue is filtered through the kidneys and excreted in the urine, energy levels naturally rise.

There are a few sea salt companies that I recommend over others: Himalayan Sea Salt, Celtic Sea Salt, and Real Salt. All three brands have a unique taste. I have found Celtic Sea Salt to be the tastiest, although the Himalayan seems to be the healthiest with over eighty minerals altogether.

Alarmingly, table salt is poisonous to the nervous system. Ninety-four percent of the world's sodium is used commercially for shellacs and abrasive cleaning agents. Table salt is created by heating up ocean salt to extract sodium chloride for its commercial use as an abrasive; whatever is left over is what you find on the typical dinner table.

When combined with the eighty-plus minerals indigenous to natural sea salt, sodium chloride is highly beneficial. When you take in sodium chloride by itself, it's a toxic poison to the body. That's why salt causes blood pressure to rise. You put a toxin in your body, and arteries immediately constrict. Your heart has to work harder, which causes blood pressure to go up.

The bottom line is that table salt will destroy your energy levels while sea salt will improve it. If you take a quarter teaspoon for every quart of water within an hour or two of rising, and on an empty stomach, it will rehydrate and detoxify you. And when you detoxify, by definition, you are increasing the energy levels of your body.

ATHLETES AND ELECTROLYTES

I work with a lot of local high school athletes, soccer players, football players, and hockey players. What I teach them gives the performance edge and hardly any sports teams know about it. Most of the athletes are drinking sports drinks, which are full of sugar, additives, preservatives, flavorings, colorings, and toxic garbage. You may get a quick shot of energy, but then you crash because the chemicals destroy blood sugar and cardiovascular performance, and eventually joints and organs. What you really want to get out of a sports drink is electrolytes, and that's what sea salt is. Pure sea salt is pure electrolytes. I teach the athletes to keep sea salt on them; liquid sea salt is best. Spray twenty or thirty spurts on your tongue, and then drink water. Bam! You're going to have endurance, stamina, strength, and power to last you as long as you need, and you'll be able to outpace the other team. That's just one of the little secrets that I teach the teams.

THE NECESSITY OF GOING ORGANIC

Organic farming methods are highly important—and not just for our individual health. Back in the 1930s, the U.S. government released a statement regarding depletion of minerals from the American soil. The concern was that the food grown in the soil at that time was seriously deficient in minerals and that new farming methods were needed. Non-organic farming methods spray plants with chemicals:

pesticides, fertilizers, herbicides, and fungicides. Consuming these chemicals has been known to cause cancer and numerous other health problems. Unfortunately, there's no quick fix because these chemicals remain in the soil and are picked up by other crops grown in it.

Organic farming methods are the solution to this problem. It's critical that, when possible, we put only organic fruits and vegetables into our bodies so that we're not taking in all these chemicals. Organic farming also preserves the eighty-plus minerals in the soil. When land is not organically farmed, it is severely depleted of minerals – sea salt minerals as well. If we're not getting those minerals, our bodies will not function properly as our cells, tissues, and organs need them. And if livestock consume nutrient-depleted grass and grains, their meat, too, will be deficient.

As of the writing of this book, the main source of produce in this country is non-organic, heavily sprayed with chemicals, and/or genetically modified. It's food that messes with our genes, can cause cancer, toxifies and acidifies our bodies, and overall makes us sick and diseased. Fortunately, organic food is becoming more affordable and more readily available. You can find good food at any local farmers markets, and now even at your neighborhood grocery store. A growing number of families are putting in small vegetable gardens in their backyard.

COCONUT OIL: GOOD FATS, BAD FATS

Polyunsaturated oils become toxic when they are oxidized as the result of exposure to oxygen, heat, or light (sunlight or artificial) causing rancidity and the formation of free radicals. Free radicals deplete our antioxidant reserves and cause chemical reactions that damage tissues and cells. When oils are extracted from seeds, they are immediately exposed to oxygen, heat, and light. The oxidation process starts even before the oil leaves the factory. The more processing the oil undergoes, the more chance it has of oxidizing. All conventional processed and refined vegetable oils are rancid to some extent by the time they reach the store. The majority of vegetable oils today, even many health food store brands, are highly processed and refined. During the refining, the oil is separated from its source with petroleum solvents and then boiled to evaporate the solvents. The oil is refined and bleached and chemical preservatives are frequently added to retard oxidation.

The safest vegetable oils to use are those processed at low temperatures and packaged in dark containers. When minimally processed, they retain most of their natural antioxidants. These antioxidants are important because they retard spoilage by slowing down oxidation and free-radical formation. The less processing that oil undergoes, the less harmful it is to the human body. Most natural oils are extracted from seeds by mechanical pressure and low temperatures, and without the use of chemicals. Oils derived by this process are referred to as expeller-pressed or cold-pressed. These are the only vegetable oils you should eat, but be careful: Even these oils are subject to oxidation and must be packaged, stored, and used properly.

Coconut oil, being a highly saturated fat, is the least vulnerable of all the dietary oils to oxidation and free radical formation and therefore is the safest to use in cooking. In addition, since it is composed primarily of medium-chain fatty acids, it is not like the long-chain saturated fatty acids that raise blood cholesterol levels. And unlike almost all saturated and unsaturated oils, it does not promote the platelet stickiness that leads to blood clot formation. Compared to other oils, coconut oil is rather benign. Replacing the liquid vegetable oils you are now using with coconut oil can help eliminate the many health problems caused by consuming oxidized oils.

While coconut oil's apparent harmlessness is a definite advantage, it is not the primary reason it is so good. The medium-chain fatty acids in coconut oil give it properties that make it unique and considered by many health practitioners to be the healthiest oil on earth.

Saturated fats are the only fats that are safe to heat and cook with. Unless the vegetable oil has been cold-pressed or expeller-pressed, it contains transfatty acids. Transfatty acids have been linked to a variety of adverse health effects, including cancer, heart disease, multiple sclerosis, diverticulitis, complications of diabetes, and other degenerative conditions.

Research has shown that medium-chain fatty acids found in coconut oil can kill bacteria and viruses that cause influenza, herpes, bladder infections, and numerous other conditions. Coconut oil is also great to use on the skin including skin rashes, eczema, psoriasis or even seriously burned or critically ill patients.

Medium-chain fatty acids are also digested and utilized differently. They are not packaged into lipoproteins and do not continue to circulate throughout the bloodstream like other fats, but are sent directly to the liver where they are immediately converted into energy just like a carbohydrate. But unlike carbohydrates, medium-chain fatty acids do not raise blood sugar, so coconut oil is safe for diabetics. Many people report that coconut oil helps them control sugar cravings and reduces hypoglycemic symptoms.

So when you eat coconut oil, the body uses it immediately to make energy rather than storing it as body fat. Therefore, you can eat much more coconut oil than other oils because the excess is not converted into fat. It has been well documented in numerous dietary studies, using animals and humans, that replacing long-chain fatty acids with medium-chain fatty acids results in a decrease in body weight gain and a reduction in fat deposition. The medium-chain fatty acids shift the body's metabolism into a higher gear so that you burn more calories. Medium-chain fatty acids increase metabolic rate, making coconut oil a dietary fat that can actually promote weight loss. Researchers at McGill University in Canada have found that if you replace long-chain triglycerides, such as soybean oil, canola oil, safflower oil, and the like, with triglycerides, such as coconut oil, you can lose up to thirty-six pounds of excess fat in a year. This is without changing your diet and without reducing the number of calories you eat; all you have to do is get an oil change!

Polyunsaturated vegetable oils depress thyroid activity, thus lowering metabolic rate. According to Ray Peat, PhD, an endocrinologist who specializes in the study of hormones, unsaturated oils block thyroid hormone secretion, its movement into circulation, and the response of tissues to the hormone. In contrast, Coconut oil stimulates metabolism, increases energy, and improves thyroid function, all of which aid in reducing unwanted body fat. The recommended dosage is three to four tablespoons per day.

SUPPLEMENTS: WHO NEEDS THEM?

More chemicals in our food are bombarding our bodies than ever before. There's more physical interference, more subluxation, and more neurological interference than ever before. Never before has there been more physical interference, more inactivity, or more sedentary lifestyles. We now have access to negativity, death, disease, and destruction on the news around the clock, and we are under more stress than ever before. Our bodies, which are also subjected to the lack of nutrients in our food, are becoming depleted rapidly and need to be supplemented. It's absolutely critical.

According to the 1992 Earth Summit, North America has the worst soil in the world. Eighty-five percent of the vital minerals have been depleted from it. People noticed this trend as far back as 1936, when the U.S. Senate issued Document 246, which said that impoverished soil in the United States no longer provided plant foods with minerals needed for human nourishment. Years and years ago, the land was able to provide us with everything we needed. Now, we're forced to supplement our bodies with vitamins.

There are different forms of supplementation, so discuss them with your chiropractor/wellness provider. A lot of my patients come to my office and say that a friend told them about vitamin B because it helps with stress. So they went to a supermarket, got a bottle of vitamin B, and started popping it. They may or may not get results, but if they do, the results may be minimal due to cheaper, lower quality nutrients. When buying vitamins, ensure that you buy quality.

"Diet-related diseases account for 68 percent of all deaths."
C. Everett Koop, former surgeon general

An apple grown in 1914 had 48 percent more calcium, 84 percent more magnesium, and 96 percent more iron than an apple has today. In 2009, we'd need to eat twenty-six apples to get the same levels as we got from one in 1914! We'd need to eat ten tomatoes to get the same amount of copper that one tomato provided in 1940.

The December 2005 *Journal of Clinical Nutrition* published a study on the nutritional value of produce, which was conducted by the Department of Agriculture from 1950 to 1999. The conclusion was that the value of our food supply has decreased by 6 to 38 percent. Nearly half the calcium and vitamin A in broccoli has disappeared; the vitamin A content in collard greens has fallen to nearly half its previous levels. Potassium dropped from 400 mg to 170 mg, and magnesium fell from 57 mg to only 9 mg. Cauliflower lost almost half its vitamin C, along with thiamine and riboflavin. The calcium in pineapple went from 17 mg to 7 mg. In June of 2002, a landmark study in the *Journal of the American Medical Association,* using thirty-six years of data, concluded that everyone needs a daily multivitamin regardless of age or health. Recent evidence has shown that inadequate levels of vitamins are risk factors for chronic diseases such as cardiovascular disease, periodontal disease, macular degeneration, osteoporosis, and many others.

It is no longer possible to avoid serious disease without supplementing. Depleted soils, premature harvesting, long transit times to market, processing, and a host of other factors have drastically reduced the nutritional quality of our food. So even the Journal of the American Medical Association now suggests every single adult should be on a very good vitamin for that very reason.

A 2002 Harvard University study reviewed 172 case-controlled nutritional studies and showed that low fruit and vegetable consumption resulted in *double the risk of cancer* for most organs including lung, pancreas, breast, and prostate. Additionally, as part of this study, 150 scientists reviewed 4,500 research studies on the relationship between nutrition and cancer. Overwhelming evidence consistently showed that fruits, vegetables, and grains could prevent cancer.

In our clinic, we provide customized nutritional recommendations for our patients. This involves measuring urine and blood chemistry to identify specific nutrient deficiencies. We then create a customized nutrition program tailored to biochemical and physiological needs. Because of the specificity, our patients achieve superior results. As we resupply the patients' nutrients, their cells become efficient instead of deficient. It is very empowering seeing patients experience dramatic transformations in their health.

The best source for a multi-vitamin is a company that I work with called Drucker Labs. They produce what I have found to be the highest quality, bio-available and absorbable, broad spectrum, liquid multivitamin on the market today. It is called Intramax. Your body can absorb a totally liquid supplement much better than a pill or capsule loaded with binders, fillers, chemical preservatives, additives, and colorings. Because it's more bio-available and your body doesn't have to break down a capsule or binder, you get far more nutrition. There are only a few vitamin labs in the world that can maintain this top level of purity and quality. Their effectiveness is amazing because they're measured for potency and numerous other standards.

There are many additional considerations required to make a high-quality vitamin supplement. One consideration is the age of the ingredients. To save money, some manufacturers use old and even outdated ingredients whose potency has diminished. How the ingredients have been shipped and stored also makes a difference. Shipping in an un-refrigerated truck in the summer or storage in a hot and humid warehouse will damage the potency. Having the mixed products sitting around prior to packaging exposes the ingredients to oxygen, moisture, and light, all of which can damage the nutrients. The packaging must be done carefully and correctly to protect the nutrients until the user consumes the product.

Manufacturers can play many games with how they list ingredients on labels. Without talking to the manufacturer and getting first-hand knowledge of what you are purchasing, it is not possible to know what is really in the pill. The first thing to look at is the type of chemical compounds that are listed for the minerals. Look at the major minerals such as calcium, magnesium, and zinc. What forms are they in? Low-quality formulas will contain cheap ingredients with low absorption rates. Here is what to avoid:

- Oxide (magnesium oxide)

- Carbonate (calcium carbonate)

- Sulfate

- Phosphate

In looking for Medium- to high-quality formulas, they will contain more expensive ingredients with maximum absorption such as:

- Aminoate

- Ascorbate

- Citrate

- Chelate

- Fumarate

- Malate

- Gluconate

- Picolinate

- Succinate

- Tartrate

A SPECIAL HIGH-ENERGY FOOD SOURCE

Avocados contain compounds that lower cholesterol and help prevent certain types of cancers, heart disease, diabetes, and obesity. Avocados have antioxidant as well as antacid properties. They contain fourteen minerals, notably iron and copper, which aid in red blood cell regeneration, and potassium. They are one of the best sources of vitamin A, contain no starch, and minimal sugar. Avocados are 80 percent fat, all of it good fat. They are a good source of protein and have more potassium than bananas without all the sugar. They are rich sources of the phytochemicals and glutathione, a powerful antioxidant and anti-aging chemical. Avocados are also the richest source of lutein, which protects against cancer and eye diseases. They are also very high in vitamin E.

Essential fatty acids are a must. Without a very specialized diet, obtaining adequate essential fatty acids is impossible. As a result, up to 90 percent of the American population may be deficient in essential fatty acids. Fats are essential to cell structure, but they must be the right kinds of fats. I strongly recommend Udo's Choice Perfected Blend Omega 3-6-9 oil product. This is an excellent daily supplement.

Antioxidant chemicals are also essential. A recent study in Free Radical Biological Medicine found that ozone in urban environments significantly reduces the amount of antioxidant vitamins in the epidermis (first layer of skin), leading to measurable free radical skin damage. A study at the Anderson Cancer Center of the University of Texas found a 70 percent drop in skin cancer risk simply by taking a daily vitamin E dose of more than 100 IU, and a 90 percent drop in skin cancer risk by taking 5,000 IU of beta-carotene. Skin damage is prevalent in cities where we have constant exposure to toxins such air and water pollutants. Because these toxins are nearly unavoidable, it is important to get adequate amounts of antioxidants such as vitamins A, C, and E, as well as carotenes and selenium. To do this, eat a diet rich in fresh fruits and vegetables, and as already mentioned, make sure it's accompanied by high-quality supplements.

LOW-ENERGY FOODS

You must avoid junk foods. They are refined, over processed, and loaded with salt, sugar, coloring, additives, and hydrogenated or partially hydrogenated vegetable oil, margarine, butter, and hidden ingredients. All refined foods are deficient, even the so-called "enriched" ones – there's a misleading term if ever there was one. Other low-energy foods include caffeinated beverages (coffee and black tea), commercialized dairy products (milk, cheese, yogurt, cream), refined wheat pasta, white rice, salt, alcohol, artificial food additives, fried foods, artificial sweeteners (such as aspartame), carbonated beverages (soft drinks), processed foods (such as white bread, crackers, bagels, pretzels, and corn).

*"Leave your drugs in a chemist's pot if you can
heal the patient with food."*
-Hippocrates

The top eight worst energy-draining foods and beverages:

1. The whites: sugar, salt, and flour

2. Doughnuts

3. French fries (and nearly all deep-fried foods)

4. Soft drinks, coffee, sports drinks, and fruit juices

5. Alcoholic beverages

6. Pasteurized dairy foods

7. Peanut butter and peanuts; most of the time they are full of mold.

8. Corn, cornstarch, and corn syrup; corn is a strong acid and should never be consumed

Energy-destroying food preparation methods to avoid:

- Microwaves

- Nonstick pans

- Frying with oils (suggestion: add healthy oils after steaming, eat food raw).

- Fast cooking of meats (better to cook foods slow).

- Boiling of vegetables (it's better to lightly steam or eat them raw).

The most toxic, energy-destroying chemicals:

- Household cleaning products

- Pesticides and herbicides

- Steroids, growth hormones, and antibiotics

- Preservatives, additives, colorings,

- hydrogenated oils, rancid fats, and other chemicals

- Teflon cookware

- Typical tap water

- Personal-care products

- Heavy metals*

- Biotoxins*

- Pharmaceuticals

HIGH-ENERGY CLEANSING

According to Dr. Isaac Jennings, "the source of disease begins with activities that drain the body of life force." One of the body's first responses to lowered nerve energy and decreased functional efficiency is the decreased elimination of waste through the lungs, respiratory tract, bowels, and urinary tract.

The body's four main filtration systems are: your liver (chemical filter), your spleen (blood cell filter), your lymphatic system (intercellular filter) and your kidneys (food filters). The body's four filtration systems need to be cleansed regularly. If not, they will sap the body of energy production. Cleansing these filters, as well as the colon is vital for health and energy levels. One of the best ways to cleanse the colon is consuming a high-fiber diet with a least thirty to thirty-five grams of fiber per day. Fiber foods are foods such as brown rice, bran, and legumes (beans and peas). Other good source of fiber include apples, pears, flaxseed, super green foods, and berries.

Four strategies for spectacular energy and health:

1. Stop poisoning and toxifying your body.

2. Cleanse and detoxify: Get it out of the system.

3. Revitalize and regenerate: provide your body with the nutrients it truly needs as has been covered extensively in this chapter).

4. Ensure maximum nerve flow through a healthy spine.

Another key is to not eat late at night. Make sure to cut your meals off early (at least three to four hours prior to bed). As I mentioned earlier, not only is this one of the keys to successful weight loss, but the energy that would normally go into the digestive process while you were sleeping, is now freed up to do the work of healing inside the neuromusculoskeletal and organ systems of your body.

"There are two great medicines: diet and self-control."

-Oscar Maximilian Bircher-Benner,
Swiss physician and nutritionist

CHAPTER SIX

EXERCISE AND PHYSIOLOGY: THE REAL VITAMIN E

*"A man's health can be judged by which he
takes two at a time —pills or stairs."*

—Joan Welsh

To express optimal health and well-being, every one of the two hundred trillion cells in your body needs a constant supply of oxygen. Oxygen is not only essential for the cells and helps produce great amounts of energy, it also sets your body up to defend itself against cancer and other degenerative diseases. Therefore, you must exercise.

Moving your body is also essential for the health of the nervous system. Your spine requires movement. Sitting all day is one of the worst things for your spine – sitting is to the spine as sugar is to the teeth. Proper movement is essential to all life. Not only does it nourish your body with oxygen, it also feeds the cerebellum through proprioceptive (movement sensation) input from the body. The combination of oxygen and proprioceptive nourishment supercharge your body's natural energy stores, enhancing health and vitality naturally. If you want a healthy brain, you have to move your body. "Ninety percent of the stimulation and nutrition to the brain is generated by the movement of the spine," notes Dr. Roger Sperry, Nobel Prize recipient for brain research. He also states, "This would be analogous to a windmill generating electricity."

Hundreds of years ago, it was common for people to walk ten, fifteen, even twenty miles a day. Today, people are reluctant to get off the couch or out of their car. And they repeat this cycle day in and day out, hardly moving their bodies.

Neurologically, two things happen as you move your body: mechanoreception and nocioception. When the spine moves, it fires off neurons called mechanoreceptors. Mechanoreceptors are like nourishment for your brain. The mechanoreceptors fire off good information to the brain as you exercise, so mechanoreception helps develop a healthy state of mind.

Here's how it works: The positive messages are fired into the cerebellum. The cerebellum is the part of the brain that controls coordination, posture, movement, intelligence, learning, and memory. The cerebellum coordinates all those functions to maximize attention span and focus. The cerebellum takes the messages it receives and fires those messages into various areas of the brain such as the amygdala, which is the stress and anxiety area, and the locus cereleus, which is another anxiety area. The cerebellum also fires messages into the hippocampus, which is the memory center, and also the hypothalamus, which is the hormone control system of the body.

If your spine is out of alignment due to subluxation, improper information is sent to the cerebellum. If you impair cerebellar development, or cerebellar plasticity, then you reduce brain-body potential. In the chiropractic profession, we are thankful for people such as Dr. James Chestnut, who has synthesized exhaustive research in the field of neurology and physiology and has done an excellent job in linking the two to performance and potential.

When you move your body and spine, it fires good messages into your cerebellum, your memory centers, your hormonal system, and your stress anxiety centers. Through exercise, stress and anxiety are reduced, and both short and long term memory is improved. Also, the hypothalamus releases good hormones that are beneficial to your whole body. The brain produces good messages that are then sent back down your spinal cord and out through the spinal nerves to all organs of the body, delivering a greater level of health, energy, and vitality.

When you don't move, your spine locks up. Muscle degeneration and neurological degeneration begins, inflammation starts to develop, and ligaments, tendons, joints, and discs begin to malfunction. Everything starts degenerating rapidly. The nerves in those areas of the spine that are locked up and subluxated start firing bad messages, or what is called nocioception, to the cerebellum. This does the exact opposite of what exercise does for you, affecting not only posture, balance, coordination, but learning, attention, focus, memory, and feelings of wellbeing. This bad information going into the cerebellum ultimately will produce disease and sickness. On a neurological level, the implications of exercise are enormous. There are few things you can do for your health that will have the phenomenal benefits that exercise does.

There are a lot of reasons people don't exercise. Mainly, they don't understand that it is vitally important for more than just weight loss. A lot of people also are fearful of going to a gym. They feel very uncertain when it comes to working out. They don't really know where to start.

Our culture actually promotes laziness. We want to make things as easy as possible and as fast as possible with as little work as possible in our quick-fix American society. Some people say they don't have time to exercise, but it doesn't take a lot of time. I'm going to share with you how to do exercise routines in as little as three or four minutes per day, three times a week, so that time is really not an excuse.

Another excuse people use for not exercising is that they don't have the energy. But remember, exercise generates energy. As exercise moves oxygen into your body, it produces positive neurological input in your brain; you're actually gaining energy. Sitting around doing nothing leaves you feeling lethargic, and that won't change until you move. Another excuse is that exercise hurts. If people already have joint pain, they don't want to move any more than they have to. But as you move your body, joints become lubricated. Oxygenation created by movement assists in transporting waste out of the joints and moving nutrients in, so the joints actually work better over time. It may be painful at first, but soon you'll be moving better and have less pain in your joints. There are few medical conditions that would make exercise a contraindication. Combining exercise with proper hydration and nutrition also contributes toward joint lubrication.

I'm certain that if people really understood all the ramifications and benefits of exercising, they'd be doing it. Not exercising makes your immune system weaker, depletes your memory and ages your brain faster, and who wants that?

TO EXERCISE OR NOT TO EXERCISE

When you don't move your body, your blood vessels become weaker and thinner. Blood pressure has to go up, because as the heart gets weaker it has to pump more times per minute to circulate the same amount of blood. When blood pressure goes up, the immune system crashes, the cells get less oxygen, and there is more chance of developing cancer. The brain is also heavily affected because it relies on heavy levels of oxygen; if it's not getting this oxygen, neurons start dying off rapidly, which is how neurodegenerative diseases such as Alzheimer's, Parkinson's, and multiple sclerosis develop, as well as a range of other mental disorders. Exercise is absolutely critical, especially for the immune system, brain function, and heart function. Exercise boosts your brain and may reverse brain decay. Research suggests that regular aerobic exercise may delay or even reverse age-related brain decline, including that associated with Alzheimer's disease and dementia. The nitric oxide that is released as a result of exercise serves as a vasodilator (artery expander), allowing the arteries to deliver greater quantities of oxygen and nutrients to the brain. According to a review of studies in the *British Journal of Sports Medicine*, "Moderate physical exercise (anything that leaves you breathless), can increase both the volume of brain tissue and the brain's ability to function."

In a study at the University of Kansas Medical Center, researchers found that patients with early Alzheimer's who worked out regularly showed less deterioration in the areas of the brain linked to memory than more sedentary patients with the disease. Other studies indicated that high levels of physical fitness have a positive effect on mental plasticity, or the brain's capacity for growth and development.

Exercise also counteracts the effects of aging, increases lifespan, and improves bone function. There is less chance of developing osteoporosis, and so as you age, your body is in better condition. Research at Penn State and Johns Hopkins reported in *USA Today* in 2004 showed that exercise was significantly more important than calcium intake for developing and keeping bones strong. One of the main causes of death in the elderly is falls that cause breakage of a hip or a bone, which then requires surgery and drugs, or can be fatal. If you're improving brain function, which exercise is proven to do, coordination is improved, so you reduce the chance of falling. If you do fall, your neuromuscular skeletal system is in better condition and you'll be able to absorb the impact of the fall and recover faster. Vestibular (balance) problems are created by interference in the central nervous system. Because falls are the leading cause of accidental death among the elderly, chiropractic care for the reduction of central nervous system interference and cerebellar (balance) health is a potential lifesaver.

EXERCISE AND LIFE-EXTENSION

Good news! Research confirms that weight training extends functional life capacity of older people. The benefit of a weight-training program has now been firmly established. After age thirty, 10 percent of muscle mass is lost every decade, however, this can be reversed with weight training. Even frail people in their nineties have gained strength and improve their mobility within a carefully monitored course of weight training. Clearly, the benefits of strength training are not limited by your age. Just like muscles, the brain adapts to a consistent exercise regime. At the University of Illinois, William Greenough determined that mice that were exercised on treadmills and taught a balancing task had more brain connections and blood vessels than mice that got significantly less exercise. This research indicates that the brain responds to physical exercise as much as any muscle does.

Could it be that exercising actually makes you smarter? University of Utah's Robert Dustman investigated electrical brain activity of elderly people, and compared an athletic group to a sedentary group. The athletic group's brain waves resembled those of younger people; the sedentary groups did not. In other words, exercising keeps you and your brain young.

Another benefit of exercise on the brain is the generation of large amounts of serotonin, the lack of which is why people take drugs such as Zoloft, Paxil, Effexor, and Prozac. Exercise naturally boosts serotonin, which improves mood and can even snap you out of depression. It improves memory, decreases anxiety, helps with cognition, increases attention and focus, and helps with learning, especially for children. Children who exercise receive all the above benefits and therefore develop and grow healthier than kids who don't. Because their brains are healthier, their bodies are healthier.

The more we exercise, the more oxygen we push into our bloodstream, the healthier we're going to be and, thus, the more energy we're going to generate. When we move, our cells get energized as they become oxygenated. Oxygen and glucose are the primary driving forces in the production of energy within a cell, so the more oxygen you can drive into a cell, the more energy you'll have.

A perfect example of this is long-distance athletes who train at higher altitudes. Their bodies acclimate to less oxygen by developing more red blood cells to help capture more oxygen. When they then compete in lower altitude atmospheres, they have more red blood cells and thus more oxygen carrying capacity in their blood, so they have more energy and endurance. Many things improve when you oxygenate the brain; brain chemistry stabilizes, and as a result you have a much healthier, better functioning brain – a whole brain, to get through life with.

"Those who think they have not time for bodily exercise will sooner or later have to find time for illness."
-Edward Stanley, former prime minister of the United Kingdom

HORMONALLY CORRECT EXERCISE

There are really two major forms of exercise: cardiovascular exercise and weight/resistance training. Cardiovascular exercise has tremendous benefits; it super oxygenates your body, strengthens your heart and blood vessels, increases HDL (good) cholesterol, and lowers VLDL ('bad') cholesterol. It also stabilizes blood sugar, improves circulation, and improves balance and vision—it even makes hair grow stronger and thicker and skin get healthier. However, there are some negatives to long-term or long stretches of cardiovascular exercise. When you exercise for an hour at a time, on average, you are adversely affecting the hormonal balance of your body. When you perform long distance exercises, your body releases negative stress hormones in the form of cortisol and catecholomines such as adrenaline, noradrenaline, and epinephrine. These hormones break down glycogen in the liver. Glycogen breaks down into glucose or sugar, which then elevates blood sugar. When blood sugar rises, insulin rises, and your body takes sugar and converts it into fat. So fat is produced when stress hormones are released. This is why a lot of marathon runners are called fat/skinny people—also known as sarcoplasmic obesity. They're thin, but they don't really have healthy muscle tone. You can make the comparison between a hundred meter sprinter and a marathon runner. Sprinters are cut, lean, and muscular. Then you look at a marathon runner, and they're just skinny, but not necessarily muscular. They're actually almost on the fat side, and some of them are clinically obese, believe it or not, because their body fat percentage is out of proportion with their muscle mass. The reason for this is the breaking down of their muscle from overuse as well as glycogen from the liver being released into the bloodstream due to the stress hormones. This results in the body producing lots of fat.

Cortisol throws off the balance of other hormones. It also stresses the immune system, so people who are long distance runners and triathletes usually have a weaker immune system due to their intense endurance training. Cortisol also negatively affects the release of growth hormone and testosterone, two key hormones for anti-aging, fat burning, muscle building, and memory. Again, there are tremendous benefits from cardiovascular exercise, however, the hormonal shift is negative and detrimental for your body.

How do you get the best of both worlds? How do you get all the advantages of cardiovascular exercise without the negative hormonal shifts? You have to add interval training. What I prescribe to my patients is three days of cardiovascular exercise and then three days of interval training (also called surge or burst training). Thirty seconds of intense effort at 90 percent maximum heart rate. To find your maximum heart rate, subtract your age from 220. Fifty to 75 percent of that number is your ideal range to burn fat during cardiovascular exercise. But, for interval training, you want thirty seconds at 90 percent of your maximum heartbeat, going as hard as you can with whatever activity that you like to do. (Only people who have no cardiovascular concerns and have been checked out by a physician should do this form of exercise. You can do interval training on a bike, swimming, rowing, cross-country, or while inline skating. A great option is racquetball or tennis; even basketball in some ways provides the quick burst of activity that also provides a degree of burst training. You can actually see the difference in the physique. Look at a basketball player. They're constantly doing bursts of exercise, so they have the right hormonal balance and their bodies are in the right physiological state: lower cortisol, higher testosterone, and higher growth hormone.

For example, if you want to ride your bike for an hour, think of when you were a kid and you would get up off the seat and pedal as hard as you could. You would do that for about twenty or thirty seconds and then start pedaling normally. After thirty seconds of coasting, you got up and did it again. A burst can be between twenty and sixty seconds, but you probably want to do it for no longer than thirty to begin with. After the initial thirty seconds, you want to be at 90 percent of your maximum heart rate. Do at least three of these thirty-second bursts with thirty-second rests in between, and insert them into your hour bike ride. When you reach 90 percent of your maximum heart rate, you're going to be breathing as hard as you can, huffing and puffing; when that happens, you're creating an oxygen debt that causes the burning up of an enormous amount of glucose, which is needed in order to put the oxygen back into your body. This also causes you to burn an enormous number of calories. The harder you breathe, the more oxygen you take into your bloodstream and the faster you burn fat. Very similar to your fireplace: The more air you give your fire, the faster it burns. I like to think of our bodies as combustion engines: the more we eat and the less we exercise, the slower the fat burns. The less we eat and more we exercise, the faster we burn and lose the fat.

Now, whatever you burn during your exercise is the exact opposite of what you will burn for the next forty-eight to seventy-two hours. If you burn a lot of sugar during the burst training, for the next couple of days, you'll be burning fat. If you're burning fat during cardiovascular training, however, you're going to be burning sugar afterward. The fastest way to train your body to burn fat is to do this type of interval training. It's the hormonally correct way of exercising, and the most powerful way of doing it is by mixing it with cardiovascular training. Again, the burst training raises your growth hormone and testosterone, decreases cortisol, and helps you burn fat faster.

You can actually mix it in with resistance or weight training as well. If you do this and a few days of cardiovascular training, you're going to keep your hormones in balance and keep all the beneficial anti-aging, health-promoting growth hormone and testosterone intact. You're going to feel great and get a lean, healthy, vital, energized body without adding fat or having trouble burning fat. When you see people in the gym, year after year, but you never really see a change in their bodies, this is why. It's not for lack of exercise; it's because their exercise is not hormonally correct. Hormonally correct exercise is the key to not only weight loss but also anti-aging, a healthy immune system, and a lean, muscular, strong, energized, vital body.

The best part: it's not expensive and anybody can do it. All you really need is a good pair of shoes and some athletic wear and you're ready to hit the pavement. You can do it with an exercise as simple as push-ups or wind sprints, and it only takes three times a week to total about twelve minutes of burst training. That's all you need to change your physiology, anatomy, how you look, and how you're burning fat. If you can combine it with another three days of cardiovascular exercise, you'll go to a whole different level of health and oxygenation of your body.

***A study from the University of New South Wales in Sydney found interval training is one of the fastest ways to shed fat. Women who spent twenty minutes mixing sprints with jogging lost three times the fat off their legs and butt in fifteen weeks than those jogging steadily for forty minutes; burn triple the fat in half the time? Bring it on!

QUICK NOTE ON RESISTANCE TRAINING

Muscles must be under continuous resistance to become stronger, leaner, and better developed. Muscles adapt to whatever force you apply to them. Or don't. If you consistently put a strain on a certain muscle group, it will adapt by getting more physically powerful, more toned, and it will change its shape. If you consistently do not put strain on your muscles, they become weaker, flabbier, and shapeless. To be healthy, lean muscle mass must increase and fat must decrease.

While aerobic exercise will cause some resistance to the set of muscles being used, it is not enough. Resistance needs to be applied throughout the entire body so you remove fat and increase leanness in all or most of the muscles. Resistance exercise occurs when you apply sustained or repetitive strain (resistance) to muscle. The most effective way to create resistance against the muscles and thus produce predictable results is a properly applied weight-lifting program. One thing I have observed in my clinical studies and research is that the healthiest and oldest people in our country lift weights. I recommend to all my patients that they join a local gym or, better yet, hire a personal trainer. This will help to get the ball rolling.

WHAT ONE POUND OF MUSCLE
CAN DO FOR YOU

One pound of muscle is thought to burn thirty-five calories per day; whereas one pound of fat burns only two calories. There are 350 calories stored in a pound of fat. If you were to gain ten pounds of muscle or lean body mass through exercise, you increase your metabolic rate by about 350 calories per day. Over a period of just 10 days, those ten new pounds of muscle will naturally burn off one pound of body fat. Even if you add only five pounds of muscle, that's 175 extra calories burned a day or eighteen pounds a year.

One way to measure health is by how much lean muscle tissue you have compared to fat tissue. Using this measurement, the more muscle you have and the less fat you have, the healthier you are. Many conditions, symptoms, and diseases are set in motion by a body with a low-muscle-to-high-fat ratio. The Tanita machine in our office provides a powerful resource for our patients since it performs and measures body fat percentages as well as body fat composition in the belly, legs, and arms. It also measures body mass index (BMI is one of the surest indicators that you will or will not develop degenerative disease), body water content, basal metabolic rate (BMR), muscle mass, fat mass, and weight. A healthy BMI is between 18.5 and 24.9. A number from 25 to 29.9 indicates a body is overweight. Any number thirty or above indicates obesity. You should also measure your waist/hip ratio. Simply measure your hip circumference at its widest part. Then measure your waist at the narrowest part of your torso. Then divide your waist measurement by your hip measurement. A healthy ratio is less than .8. The ideal ratio is .74. If your ratio is greater than .85, you are at risk for many health conditions. Another important measurement is your body fat percentage. Body fat percent for men between 10 to

18 percent is considered healthy. A body fat percentage between 20 and 28 is considered healthy for women in their peri-menopausal or menopausal years, while 12 to 23 percent is ideal for younger women. Women need to reduce body fat to below 20 percent to strongly reduce their risk of breast cancer

TOXICITY AND EXERCISE: HOW TO REMOVE STRESS, CHEMICALS, AND NEUROTOXICITY WHILE GETTING YOUR VITAMIN E

Neurotoxicity such as heavy metal toxicity from vaccines, amalgam fillings, pesticides, herbicides, and other chemical residues as well as biotoxins such as household molds alters your metabolic control center (the hypothalamus) causing weight gain, low energy, and hormonal fluctuations. We're exposed to toxic man made chemicals from everyday items such as magazines, newspapers, carpets, pillows, mattresses, clothes, cosmetics, toothpaste, and processed foods. Toxic chemicals are responsible for many of our 20th century disease problems and especially the new syndromes that leave doctors scratching their heads. Fatigue, headaches, digestive issues, "flu-like" symptoms, and aching joints can all be caused by environmental chemicals. High blood pressure and even fatal cardiac arrhythmias can be caused by chemicals ranging from solvents to pesticides. People who wake up feeling sluggish may not realize that the cause is right under their nose in the polyester chemicals being emitted from their own pillow.

We live in a soup of toxicity and we'll never completely escape it, but exercise will help with natural toxin elimination. Exercise, your natural vitamin E, is one of the best ways to sweat these toxins out of your system.

Another great form of detoxification exercise is rebounding. Rebounding (or "trampolining") is also known as cellular exercise. Every cell in the body is simultaneously stimulated and strengthened while jumping on the rebounder. This unique form of exercise dramatically increases the movement of the lymph system, increases oxygen to the cells, releases tension and stress, stimulates every cell toward elimination of toxins, and increases the strength and vitality of every cell in the body.

Whole body vibration (WBV) therapy and endocrinology (see appendix for ordering information) is available at Yachter Family Chiropractic Center. WBV is another effective way to both detoxify as well as hormonally balance your body. WBV decreases levels of cortisol (again, commonly referred to as the stress hormone), which is found in elevated levels in cancer patients. Cortisol increases the build-up of fatty tissue in the body, catabolizes (breaks down) muscle mass into free amino acids, and increases levels of blood sugar. WBV has been shown to increase levels of human growth hormone by up to 361 percent. This hormone accelerates the anabolism (synthesis) of protein to stimulate growth and regeneration, and breaks down fat into fatty acids, providing a boost in energy levels. Some people pay for injections of synthetic human growth hormone, commonly referred to as the anti-aging hormone, at a cost of a few thousand dollars per shot in an attempt to combat and reverse the effects of aging. WBV therapy also has been shown to increase levels of testosterone, which plays key roles in the health and well-being of both males and females by enhancing libido, energy, immune function, and protecting against osteoporosis. It also increases muscles mass and strength, as well as bone density. Testosterone levels decline gradually with age, which may cause infertility, decreased libido, erectile dysfunction, osteoporosis, loss of appetite, and/or anemia.

LOOK HOW EASY THIS IS!

Walk about one and a half miles each day and get fit:

Aerobic capacity: 19% increase

Physical function: 25% increase

Risk of disability: 41% decrease

Save on annual medical bills

Normal-weight retiree saves: $3,300

Overweight retiree saves: $2,500

Entire country saves: $1.4 trillion

Improve cardiovascular health

Heart disease: 32% lower risk

Stroke: 33% lower risk

Type 2 diabetes: 71% lower risk

Fight cancer

Breast: 18% lower risk

Colon: 31% lower risk

All forms: 33% higher survival rate

Lose weight

Each walk: 150 calories

Monthly: 1.3 pounds

Annually: 15.6 pounds

Accelerate recovery

Depression: 47% reduction of symptoms

Skin wounds: Shorten healing by 10 days

Battle degenerative disease

Alzheimer's: 40% lower risk

Arthritis: 46% lower risk

Osteoporosis: Zero loss of bone density

ACCOUNTABILITY

I'm a big fan of accountability in all aspects of my life—financially, professionally, and in relationships. In everything I do, accountability keeps me on my toes. If I commit to exercise and somebody is waiting for me to workout, then I know that I'm not going to let that person down; I'm going to show up. I'm more likely to stick with that program I've established and reach my goals if I have somebody there pushing me to follow through, and vice versa. Accountability is crucial to achieving your goals.

Again, before starting your exercise program, you need to make sure that you do not have any of the following issues: hypertension, arthritis, heart disease, dizzy spells, inability to take on mild forms of physical exertion without leading to a breathless state, previous history of ligament and muscle tears, or currently taking prescription drugs. The health risks are minimal when a person in good health engages in physical activity. They are also minimal when you follow the advice of your health practitioner. On the contrary, excessive periods of inactivity, bad nutrition habits, spinal subluxation, and overeating all present health risks that are far greater.

CHAPTER SEVEN

STRESS MANAGEMENT: TAME TODAY, TRANSFORM TOMORROW

"If you do not conquer self, you will be conquered by self." —Napoleon Hill

Today we live in a more stressful environment than ever. Just turn on the news. There's more crime. There's more rage. There's more anger. There's more violence. There's more war. There's more rape, murder, and theft than ever before. Even the positive aspects of our lives create stress: We're always on the phone, in the car, at work, and we never seem to have time to relax. We rush around more today than ever; stress seems to be the biggest killer. Conservative medical experts generally agree as much as 75 percent of human illness is stress-related. Excessive, uncontrolled stress can ravage our immune systems, leaving our bodies susceptible to attack. We definitely need to learn how to take control of our day; if we don't take control, it will take control of us.

How do you get your life in order? It's all about prioritizing; understanding first and foremost what's most important. Then you must make sure that you give the most attention and focus to those things. In our office we have people break down the most important aspects of their lives: relationships with family and friends, relationship with God, professional life, personal life, etc. Then we ask them to identify what their priorities are. That's what we call priority living, or value management.

A lot of patients ask if it's really possible to manage stress, and the answer is an unequivocal yes. You can do this by keeping your life in order so you don't have breakdowns mentally and physically. Instead of managing stress, you're actually managing energy and expenditure of it before things get chaotic. We teach our patients to focus on energy management, not time management. Your body and mind are like a battery, and the energy it contains must be protected and renewed regularly. The way we do this is by focusing energy into things that are worthy and worthwhile.

"Goals provide the energy source that powers our lives. One of the best ways we can get the most from the energy we have is to focus it. That is what goals can do for us: concentrate our energy."
-Denis Waitley, motivational coach

Focused mental and emotional energy is a characteristic trait not only of healthy individuals, but of top performers as well. Top performers manage their stress and maintain order in their lives based on priorities. They put first things first. Low performers, by contrast, wake up without priorities and without a plan. They know they have things to do, but they don't have them written down. There is no real order to the day, thus draining them of their focus and their energy. Most people only have a list of things in their heads. Some people improve on this and actually write the list down. They have all these different tasks just sprinkled on a piece of paper with no rhyme or reason, no logic, no order, just a whole bunch of things that they need to do. Others manage to put the list of things they want to accomplish in a Palm Pilot, calendar, or day planner. Believe it or not, that's still a low-level way of doing things. In the fourth tier, the high-performance tier, where you manage your day and not vice versa, you'd actually have blocks of time mapped out. These are the tasks and priorities that are of top value to you, your family, and your mission that you wish to fulfill personally or professionally, and these roles are how you structure your week.

Let's take exercise as an example. The fitness component of your life is absolutely fundamental to being healthy. So you commit to exercising the six days a week that we talked about first thing in the morning, which is the most likely time that you're going to exercise and stick to it. You say, "I'm going to exercise from 6 to 6:30, Monday through Saturday, six days a week, and I'm totally committed to it." What you do next is chisel that time out: that half-hour segment of time becomes a part of your life that's immovable. It doesn't matter if someone asks you to schedule a meeting or you have to catch up on your work or even sleep. Nothing interferes with that time. You're not going to put something from your "to do" list in there; you're not going to read a book during that time. Other tasks can't fit into that block of time, because that block is already filled up. Why? Because it's a priority and an activity that you highly value.

Another highly valued time might be relationship time. Instead of haphazardly hoping to get relationship time in during the week, you might plan that every Friday night and all day Sunday is your relationship time with your family. If you violate that time by trying to squeeze in an unrelated "to-do" list activity or staying late at work, then the health of your family relationship will suffer. Sunday might also include spiritual time that doesn't get violated, meaning you don't do other things. Once you put these value times in where nothing can cross over, they're set in stone. If someone calls you for a meeting on Friday night at 6:30, you know your answer is no. You can't do it because that time is already set aside; that's priority time. Other tasks don't elbow out your priority time.

Dr. Stephen Covey, author of *7 Habits of Highly Effective People*, calls this managing the big rocks, the pebbles, and the sand. First to go into the bucket are the big rocks, which are your priorities or top values. Then your tasks (your pebbles) and then your sand (miscellaneous, trivial activities, non-mission based, time-wasting events) fill in the gaps between the big rocks. This is how top performers manage their top values and their lives. They know what's important to them and what's not, and they conduct their lives and their days as such.

STRESS CONTROL AND ENERGY MANAGEMENT

*"The key to success is to focus our conscious mind on things
we desire, not things we fear."*
-Brian Tracy, author and motivational speaker

If we allow stress to drain our minds of energy, there is a psychosomatic connection that results in a negative affect on our bodies. Just by thinking stressful thoughts, your body produces negative hormones. When you think negative thoughts or experience stress on a regular basis, several things happen. There is an increased production of cortisol and catecholamines, which do all the negative things we talked about earlier. Again, the body in response to stress produces cortisol. It is a catabolic (break-down) hormone when produced in more than needed quantities (occurs with chronic exposures to high levels of stress). Cortisol, in large quantities, will destroy or ferment skeletal muscle. Cortisol is also known as "the death hormone." When floating around the bloodstream in large quantities, cortisol signals to the body that it is time to spontaneously end its own life. These stress hormones also cause inflammation, weight gain, and fatigue. When you think thoughts, stress hormones that are being released cause your body to expend tremendous amounts of energy. So, if you want to control the amount of energy you have, it's absolutely essential that you control the way you process and perceive the stressful events that may be occurring in your surroundings.

Stress is not a tangible thing. It's not concrete. You can't reach into a bucket and grab a handful of it. In fact, if two people are in the same situation, one can interpret it as an incredibly stressful event while the other remains relaxed or unaffected. So, stress in itself is not something that's tangible; there are only stressful thoughts and how we respond to those thoughts.

A perfect example of this is in the book *Man's Search for Meaning*, by Dr. Victor Frankl, who was a Holocaust survivor. After he was liberated, Frankl decided to put a different meaning on his suffering. Instead of hating the Nazis and cursing God and humanity, he decided to live his life with forgiveness, peace, and understanding. He used that experience to develop a whole new branch of psychology and psychiatry known as logotherapy. He took this horrific nightmare experience of being in the Dachau and Auschwitz concentration camps and turned it around for good.

This is an extreme case, to be sure. Concentration camps produced some of the highest stress conditions possible. Many people committed suicide after they had been freed because they couldn't handle the terrible mental and physical stress their experience caused them. Many others retreated into bitterness and anger that affected their future relationships because they could not come to peace with such an injustice. Certainly this is understandable, even likely. But Dr. Frankl exemplifies that stress can be a matter of thought control. If Dr. Frankl could control his stress, we can certainly try to do the same. It's a matter of how we interpret things and how we process actual events and environments.

The physiological effects of stress are numerous. Several areas of the brain are engaged when it processes your environment as stressful. We've talked about the amygdala and the locus cereleus. These are the two anxiety and stress centers of the brain that are engaged by your thoughts. When you're under stress or when you interpret things as stressful, those two areas of your brain fire off into your hypothalamus and hippocampus, with multiple results.

The hippocampus is the memory and learning center. When you're under a lot of stress, your ability to remember things short-term and long-term are affected. It becomes difficult to learn and difficult to concentrate. The hypothalamus controls the release of hormones. Stress causes it to release a negative cascade of hormones throughout your body. As you now know, all these hormones have side effects such as raised blood pressure and cholesterol and increased blood sugar, which can ultimately lead to heart disease, stroke, and diabetes. You gain weight and you start burning out organs. For example, the kidneys get stressed because of the amount of blood sugar and hormones they have to deal with. The liver gets stressed because it has to work overtime to detoxify the body. And on top of all that, negative hormones affect the brain. Everything starts breaking down because of all the blood sugar; which combines with proteins in the skin, and causes your skin to age. If the blood sugar combines with the proteins of your eye, it can be a cause of cataract formation. It causes hardening of the arteries, athero-sclerosis, and arterial sclerosis. The list of physiological effects goes on and on.

STRESS CAUSES BRAIN DAMAGE

When those hormones I mentioned a moment ago are released, glucose is diverted away to the brain to fuel it for the "fight" or "flight" response. Once your brain and your senses are sharpened and prepared for "battle", the glucose is diverted from your brain to your muscles and your skeleton. When this happens, it actually causes brain damage, because your brain gets deprived of glucose/sugar. The impact of the adrenaline hitting the hippocampus, one of the parts of the brain involved with learning and memory, is severe. These stress hormones kill neurons upon contact. They actually destroy the gray matter of the central nerve system.

So, you can now see the damaging effect of stress on people. They may be running marathons, eating organic, raw foods, yet still have heart attacks, cancer and neurodegenerative disease and die young. Stress is "eating them alive." It has been shown through research that cancer often forms in the human body after the loss of a loved one, or a divorce. The mind/body connection is powerful. It immediately affects you on some level. That's why it's critical to keep stress in check.

QUESTIONS HELP CONTROL STRESS

Over nine years ago, I decided to build my own chiropractic clinic. I drove around Central Florida exploring and researching various locations in which I'd like to live. I eventually dropped anchor in Lake Mary (twenty minutes north of Orlando). As I originally drove through the town of Lake Mary, I felt that it was destiny. It was a spiritual experience. I heard a voice that told me this is where I was going to practice. I knew nobody in Lake Mary, and I had never even been in this town before. But, I went out to build a practice.

I had never built a practice before. I had never built a business before or even opened an office. I was about to experience a very traumatic journey.

One of the first issues I had to deal with was obtaining a building permit in order to do construction work. This was all very new to me. I went down to the county and submitted my building permit. I thought I'd get the approved permit returned to me within two or three weeks which would enable me to start building. It was a relatively small space that I was renting, nothing major. One month later, I still didn't have the building permit. A few months passed, and still no permit. Now I'm really starting to sweat. Three months pass and I'm ready to go bankrupt before I even open my doors. From this experience, I ended up having a panic/anxiety attack. It wasn't anything I'd call fun. It was like a ton of bricks sitting on my chest all day long. I couldn't even breathe. In my head I kept saying "If I don't get my building permit,

I'm going to crash." I was running out of money and was desperate to start my practice. I kept focusing on "the wall." What happens if this happens, what happens if that happens? I kept asking negative questions as I was headed toward crashing into that wall. Finally one morning, I awoke to my heart racing at about 300 beats a minute, feeling as if I were having a heart attack. It was then I resolved to find a solution.

This was a breaking point for me. I said, "I'm going to start asking different questions." I'd just been spinning my wheels. I started asking, "What do I need to do today to get my building permit?" I started asking myself where could I get positive answers to help me reach my destination. I went down to the county and found a Mr. Goldman, one of the directors of permits and a very helpful man. I went right up to him and said, "Listen, what do I need to do to walk out of your building with a permit in my hand?" It was a very specific question. "What do I need to do today to walk out the front door with a permit?" He told me exactly what I needed to do. Believe it or not, I got a permit that same day! I stopped looking at the wall and I looked in the direction in which I wanted to go. I got resourceful. It was as simple as that. Until then, I hadn't seen how easy it was because I'd been swept away in a sandstorm of confusion, fear, anxiety, and I wasn't asking the right questions. I was looking at the wall, but thank God I moved away from it.

What happens when you get into a stressful situation? Asking the right questions is one of the best ways to get out of a tailspin. This is how race-car drivers are taught to avoid a crash when they find themselves spinning out of control toward the wall. They know that they first have to look away from the wall. When they do, the steering wheel, and thus the tires, and the car's direction, will follow. Questions allow you to avoid "hitting the wall" and allow you to start moving in a healthy and empowering direction. The answers always come when you begin asking the right questions. If you continue to think as you have always thought, you'll continue to get as you've always gotten. Albert Einstein said, "You cannot solve the present problems at the same level the problem existed when the problem was first created." If you keep asking the same questions, your body responds. Your body chemistry responds to your thoughts and questions. It's essential to understand what stress does to the body.

Questions to ask yourself daily to minimize the effects of stress and optimize your energy potential:

1. How will the food that I'm about to eat make me feel in two hours/the rest of the day?

2. Will the food choices that I'm making create energy or lethargy and sickness in my body?

3. Will sitting on the couch and not beginning my exercise program affect my future?

4. How will neglecting my health affect my family?

5. How will my health choices affect my relationships?

6. How will the medications that I am taking affect my body if I continue to use them long-term?

7. How will the medications I am taking eventually impact my organs?

8. What will happen in the future if I don't correct my subluxations?

9. What may be happening right now if my heart, thyroid, and other organs are not receiving the proper nerve supply from my brain because of subluxation?

10. What is interfering with allowing me to experience maximum peace and joy?

The secret to maintaining your energy level is to always focus on the things you can control and not waste your time, energy and power on the things you can't control. In other words, focus on solutions, not problems. What can we control? Ourselves!

One way to achieve this is to focus on solutions and develop personal resources. If we only focus on what we can control, we'll be much happier. We can control our thoughts and actions. But focusing on the things we can't change is very energy draining. People with a positive attitude who always have chosen to focus on solutions are not only happier and more successful in all aspects of life, but they also are much healthier.

STRESS AND DRUGS

Another effect of the stress response is that the brain utilizes an enormous amount of serotonin. Stress affects the amygdala and the locus cereleus, and those two parts of the brain negatively inhibit the production of serotonin. When serotonin levels drop, the old medical way of fixing it is to prescribe serotonin-producing drugs, selective serotonin re-uptake inhibitors (S.S.R.I.). These drugs artificially boost the serotonin in the brain. These medications cause the brain's ability to make serotonin malfunction; the patient is unable to come off the drug because the brain now doesn't make normal levels of serotonin. This is called "negative feedback." This is why the natural ways of keeping stress down are so important. Like I have mentioned earlier in the book, many studies have shown that walking three times per week for thirty minutes works better than taking antipsychotic and antidepressant medications There have even been studies that show increased likelihood of suicide and violence while taking medications like these. Many school shooting since the Columbine High School shootings has been perpetrated by a person who had taken a psychotropic medications. More than thirty million Americans—one in every ten—have taken an antidepressant. Side effects include neurological disorders, such as disfiguring facial and whole-body tics that can indicate brain damage; sexual dysfunction in up to 60 percent of users; debilitating withdrawal symptoms (including visual hallucinations), electric shock-like sensations in the brain, dizziness, nausea, and anxiety; and a decrease of antidepressant effectiveness in about 35 percent of long-term users. The news is equally bad for other drugs that seek to control the symptoms of a stressful life. When stress pushes your blood pressure up, the old medical solution is to prescribe medications that push your blood pressure down. And it will go down, but you still have your problem because the stress is still there. The cause is not gone; one of its symptoms has just been quieted. The body's innate mechanisms are going to keep trying to push the blood pressure up, and if you try to come off your medication, your blood pressure will often go even higher than it was before.

In our office, I am committed to working with patients who have made a personal decision to find the source of their problem and improve their health naturally, doing whatever it takes. I've witnessed thousands of people come off blood pressure medications, antidepressants, and many other types of medications after discovering the true cause of their problem, and I've never seen one person do so and not be healthier. I'm not saying that such medications are never needed, but I've never seen one person who didn't get healthier once they identified and addressed the true cause of their problem. Obviously, as I have mentioned, there are exceptions; one being the person who is either missing organs or has had them surgically altered.

Current scientific research is beginning to demonstrate that it's extremely dangerous to lower cholesterol artificially. When I took my degree at the University of Florida in nutrition, the first thing I learned in Nutrition 101 was that if you want to get someone healthy, you have to get their bloodstream as clean as possible. The second thing we were taught is that heart disease is not caused by cholesterol. It never has, and never will. It's caused by high blood sugar, which elevates hormones such as insulin and raises triglycerides. That's what clogs your arteries. We should remember: High cholesterol is a symptom that is produced in response to high levels of stress. Medical doctors have known for over a decade that 50% of people who have a heart attack do not have elevated cholesterol levels.

Dr. Uffe Ravnskov, MD, PhD, who wrote the book The Cholesterol Myths, reviews study after study debunking the idea that high cholesterol levels are the cause of heart disease. In the Framingham Heart Study, the largest heart study ever conducted, done near Boston that spanned 30 years and involved over 15,000 patients, researchers concluded that high cholesterol was a risk factor for heart disease, but when one really dissects the data, one must question how they came to that conclusion. For example, when the participants of the study are plotted on a graph it clearly shows that those with cholesterol levels between 182 and 222 did not survive as long as those with higher cholesterol levels of between 222 and 261. The study shows that approximately half the people with heart disease had low cholesterol, and half the people without heart disease had high cholesterol.

When you're under a lot of stress cholesterol is very important. It's there to protect you and is a natural antidepressant, and it calms your brain down. If you're under a lot of stress and take cholesterol-lowering medications, the drug lowers the cholesterol from your brain and you can become depressed. That's why we're seeing a worldwide issue with individuals committing suicide while taking statin (cholesterol lowering) drugs, because cholesterol is innately designed to protect you. At least 90 percent of the population could eat a five-egg omelet with yolk intact five times per day, and their cholesterol levels wouldn't budge. The reason: The liver makes cholesterol and acts like a cholesterol thermostat. When you ingest more cholesterol, your liver produces less. When you take in less cholesterol, your liver then makes more. It makes sure that the cholesterol level is balanced. So it's never really a problem for the majority of people. When your body is healthy and the effects of stress are minimized, blood tests will naturally demonstrate a lower cholesterol level. The healthiest individuals under regular chiropractic care in my office have cholesterol levels ranging from 120-170mg/dl.Again, acidic sugar and foods that metabolically break down into sugar, and the havoc they wreak once they enter the bloodstream, are the real issue.   Very few people know that it was Big Pharma that initially established 240 as the normal cholesterol level. They set that number for a reason. The actuaries and statisticians understood that 25 percent of the American population had a cholesterol level over 240. So they figured they could create a market for at least that 25 percent of the population. Several years later, they lowered it from 240 to 220, and later lowered it to 200, where it is today. By doing that, they qualified another thirty-six million people to take these statin drugs.

Many of the popular cholesterol-lowering drugs have been linked to strokes, cancer, heart disease, and death from heart attacks.

Here's why heart attacks could be possible. A nutrient called coenzyme Q10 works like diesel fuel to power your cells. It produces energy. Your heart muscle produces pumping power off coenzyme Q10. Statin drugs can strip the CoQ10 out of your body, including your heart. That's why people taking these drugs seem to have more heart attacks than people who don't. People who take these statin drugs actually have more heart attacks than people who have "high" cholesterol and take nothing at all. It is a known fact that at least half of all people who have a heart attack or die from heart disease have normal cholesterol. Cholesterol lowering medications lower cholesterol, but you just die faster, so it doesn't make a difference. Lying in a casket with low cholesterol is not a desirable clinical outcome!

Again, there is an innate healing mechanism which produces more cholesterol and raise blood pressure when you're under a lot of stress. By removing the stress, you remove the symptoms; to do so artificially is just replacing one problem with several other severe problems.

The most natural ways of relieving the stress effects are receiving chiropractic adjustments, eating cleaner plant-based foods, putting fewer chemicals in your body, exercising, and focusing your mind in a positive direction.

THE ART AND SCIENCE OF BALANCING

Stress management is the art and science of balancing, not eliminating the nearly limitless supply of "stressful events" in our daily lives. When stress becomes our master, we quickly see its manifestation: the executive who's too stressed out to make profitable decisions; salespeople too stressed out to make convincing presentations; parents too stressed out to control kids. In every case it wasn't too much stress that did the damage, it was too little recovery or balancing. Here's a key point: Without enough quality food, water, and sleep, we're all losers. As the great coach of the Green Bay Packers football team, Vince Lombardi, once said, "fatigue makes cowards of us all." Success in every field of human endeavor requires adequate recovery. If we are to perform at our best, we must make sure we have included nonvigorous activities throughout our week.

The following activities will allow us to recapture and recover lost mental and emotional energy: walking, yoga, meditation, stretching, Tai Chi, fishing, activities such as golf, swimming, hiking, jogging, biking, and tennis. Take fifteen or twenty minute breaks every ninety to 120 minutes, particularly during periods of high physical, mental, or emotional stress. Take afternoon naps whenever possible, get seven to eight hours sleep every twenty-four hours (carefully monitor sleep activities during periods of high stress). If possible, establish the cycle of going to bed early between ten and midnight and getting up early between six and eight in the morning. Monitor your sense of fun and enjoyment daily. When you're having fun, you're literally recharging your mental battery, and at the same time recovering emotional energy.

Always have a nourishing breakfast. Limit three mental and emotional energy destroyers from your diet: alcohol, which is a depressant; caffeine, which can leave you physically and mentally drained; and sugar. After giving you a burst of energy, sugar causes a let-down, which will leave you tired and depressed. Consume some form of complex, alkalizing carbohydrates every two to four hours (four to five servings of fruit and vegetables daily). If you're overly acidic, it makes you susceptible to many ailments including headaches, chronic illnesses, colds and flu, digestive problems, urinary tract infections, and chronic fatigue. Particularly during periods of high stress it is recommended that you drink half your body weight in ounces of water each day. ie. a 180 lb. person should aim for 90 ounces of water each day or approx. 3 qts. The more water rich foods we eat, the less water we need to drink; the more concentrated the food selections, the more water you need to drink.

EXERCISE AND DEPRESSION

Exercise has even been found to be a viable alternative to traditional medical treatment of depression. In a study involving eighty adults ages twenty to forty-five who were diagnosed with mild to moderate depression, researchers looked at exercise alone to treat the condition and found that depressive symptoms were cut almost in half after twelve weeks in those individuals who participated in thirty-minute aerobic exercise sessions three to five times a week. The results of this study prove that not all patients need to rely on drugs to treat depression. Why isn't the public being told that exercise and sugar pills work just as well, if not better, than mind-altering medications? No drug that I know of on the market can make a 50 percent improvement in a person with depression. Not one.

As I've mentioned throughout this book, everything goes back to the spine, including stress. When you're under a lot of stress, everything locks up. Stress messages coming from your brain constrict and lock the muscles, ligaments, and tendons. As soon as the spine is constricted and stressed out, it starts firing bad messages back into the brain, which result in sickness and dis-ease. Stress can be relieved, first of all, when you adjust the spine. This is why chiropractic adjustments are vital and essential to stress management. Adjusting the spine helps relieve pressure off the spinal cord and nerves. This sends beneficial, advantageous, positive electrical messages up into the brain. When positive messages reach those parts of the brain, the brain produces beneficial chemicals. That healthy physiology spreads its effect over the entire body. Every organ and every tissue cell is positively affected by a chiropractic adjustment. When I adjust the spine, specifically the cervical area, most of my patients tell me they feel relaxed and a sense of euphoria. There is a specific biochemical high from the adjustment. I know from my personal experience of receiving chiropractic care for over twenty years, that immediately following every adjustment, my lungs open up, my energy significantly improves, I can breathe better, my heart works better, and my vision clears. When the upper cervical area is adjusted, massive quantities of feel-good chemicals are released in the body. Among these neuropeptides are endorphins, which are opiate-type chemicals. This is one way the chiropractic adjustment positively affects the brain/body communication.

MENTAL HEALTH AND CHIROPRACTIC

The early twentieth century saw the establishment of several inpatient mental health facilities where chiropractic adjustments were the dominant clinical service. Two of these were in Davenport, Iowa. In 1922, the Chiropractic Psychopathic Sanitarium was established. The facility was later known as Forest Park Sanitarium. North Dakota Judge A.W. Ponath noted that at the North Dakota State Mental Hospital, the "cure and discharge rate" ranged from 18 to 27 percent, compared with 65 percent at Forest Park. The second facility, Clear

View Sanitarium, was established in 1926. In 1951, the Palmer School of Chiropractic acquired Clear View. Dr. W. Heath Quigley, who directed the sanitarium, described clinical protocol: "Each day, each patient was examined with the neurocalometer (NCM). If the clinician interpreted the NCM to indicate nerve impingement (subluxation), the patient was adjusted." Quigley reported that the rooms were "sunny and bright" and that meals included "large servings of fresh vegetables from a garden."

Dr. Hayek reported at the international conference on spinal manipulation that his recent study in Australia showed that chiropractic care significantly decreased cortisol levels, anxiety levels and depression levels, and significantly increased immune function. Dr. Hayek reported that only the group undergoing spinal adjustments displayed significant improvement in asthma symptoms and depression and anxiety scores. In addition, patients actually undergoing spinal adjustments displayed dramatic increases of IGA (immune system booster) and decrease of cortisol through the post-treatment.

How does this happen? Subluxations (which create deficient nerve supply) such as forward head posture, loss of cervical curve, and lateral deviations in the spine (scoliosis) put tremendous stress on the brain-body connection, affecting every organ in the body including the thyroid, adrenals, and gut. This causes numerous pathological consequences in the body including, among others: poor nutrient absorption, metabolic irregularities, brain chemistry imbalances, poor sleep, weight gain and fatigue.

"LIFE ISN'T ABOUT HOW TO SURVIVE THE STORM,
BUT HOW TO DANCE IN THE RAIN."

THE ONE-HUNDRED-YEAR MINDSET

I try to maintain the one-hundred-year mindset and encourage my patients to do the same. The fundamental question of that mindset is, "What am I doing today that's going to allow me to live every year the human body is capable of?" Scientifically and biblically, we know that the body is built to live at least 120 years. And reaching one hundred doesn't mean sitting in a nursing home wearing diapers and drooling on myself or taking twenty medications. I'm talking about having quality of life when you reach one hundred, which is possible. The only way it's possible is if you start asking yourself what do I need to do now so I can reach that goal. That's the one-hundred-year mindset. "What is it that I'm doing second by second, minute by minute, hour by hour, day by day, month by month, week by week, and year by year?" This is what it takes if you want to join "The Century Club."

A lot of people think, "I don't want to live life that way. That's just too much thinking for me" or " everybody is going to die someday anyway, why work that hard?" Well, think about this: 90 to 95 percent of all Americans end up suffering. By the time they are sixty-five they will be on thirteen medications and if you asked any of those people if they could go back and do it differently, most say they'd give any amount of money and give any part of their life to do so.

So while it may be tedious to think about, it's imperative that you invest your time and your days properly, because right now approximately one out of one thousand people in our country makes it to age sixty without taking any medications. There's something wrong with that, and if we're going to change, we have to do it now. Remember, if you are sixty or seventy and already in that situation, it can be turned around. Implementing a new lifestyle and living the wellness culture that we have introduced to you in this book can change it. It is possible to turn it all around, and it all has to do with the one-hundred-year mindset.

Another factor in this equation is friendship. If you're going to live to be one hundred, you'll want to do it with a network of friends and family. Friends not only offer companionship but also a support network of love, which helps to reduce stress. Having a social network of friends and family with whom you can talk and express emotions and feelings is a great stress reliever. People who listen to you, who are close to you, trust you, believe in you and really care about you add to your health profile.

It's been proven that people living the longest, healthiest, happiest lives have strong social stimulation. They have lots of good friends and a lot of family around them. They're usually happy, healthy people. Their mindsets are very different. The people who live to be one hundred exhibit a positive, loving mindset. This trait is more common and important than any other single health factor. It's their psychological vantage point, how they see the world; and seeing the world as a nice place tends to make you want to hang around longer.

I've taken care of patients in their nineties and older. The people who make it that long do a lot of important things for their health. A lot of them eat very well. A lot of them exercise. A lot of them get adjustments. The most common thread that is weaved through all of their lives is that they process stress differently than others. They're calmer. They're more relaxed. They let stress roll off them. They don't take things too seriously. They ask the questions like, "Is it really worth it for me to get upset about this? Is it worth it for me to ruin a lifetime relationship? Is it worth it for me to get into a stressful situation? Is it worth it to me not to forgive this person? Is it worth it to get angry, to hold a grudge? Is this a big enough issue in the grand scheme of things, in a hundred-year lifespan? In the grand scheme of things, will it matter in twenty, fifty, or seventy years what's happening to me right now?

Asking these questions continually and habitually is one of the factors that I've found really helps these people stay calm, "manage" stress, manage their state of mind, and control the events rather than letting the events control them.

"Learn to differentiate between what is truly important
and what can be dealt with at another time."

—Mia Hamm, Olympic soccer champion

DON'T WORRY, BE HAPPY!

According to motivational speaker Zig Ziglar, here is a reliable estimate of the things people worry about: Things that never happen, 40 percent; things that can't be changed by all the worry in the world, 30 percent; needless worries about our health, 12 percent; needless worry, 10 percent; and real, legitimate worry, 8 percent. In short, 92 percent of a typical person's worry takes up valuable time, creates painful stress, and is unnecessary.

CHAPTER EIGHT

A NEW VISION FOR AMERICA

"It's been said that the only constant is change.
I don't agree with that. There's another constant,
and that's the desire for change."
-Dr. Robert Maurer, Kaizen expert, psychologist

My vision is to see a paradigm shift in America's healthcare; and I believe it all starts with families, primarily the next generation. I want to see children growing up understanding God's laws of health and healing and the way he truly designed the body to function and heal. Our body is a self-healing organism, and we carry within ourselves this innate healing ability that we can put our faith in and rely upon. It can restore us to health and wholeness if we just allow it to do so without interference.

I want people to understand the premise of the three major interferences and to know that if we can remove those interferences, the body can heal itself and get well. We must remove the chemical interferences, the physical interferences, and the emotional/psychological interferences and allow the body to express itself from above, down, inside, and out — from the brain and nervous system (the master control system), through the brain/body connection, out through the spine, and to the body.

My vision is that people get out of the pill, potion, lotion, spoonful-of-medicine mentality and start putting their faith in their own bodies, and in God's laws of health and healing. Digging ourselves out of the hole we're in starts with this belief in the body.

A wellness coach can help you begin living this lifestyle. It is paramount that you find someone to hold you accountable and provide you with the resources to begin living this lifestyle. Ideally, this person will create an atmosphere that is supportive, nurturing, encouraging, inspiring, and exciting. That person needs to show you that they are willing to hold you accountable, have ways to measure and demonstrate your progress, and ultimately be able to produce results while leading you to where you need to be. The most qualified people for this are family and wellness oriented chiropractors because they understand this philosophy and possess and utilize the resources necessary to produce outstanding results. They understand how God made the body, as well as how He heals the body; they understand His laws of health and healing.

Many remember the following story of Professor Pausch. Randy Pausch was a Carnegie Mellon computer professor who died recently from pancreatic cancer. He is a perfect example of what happens when people don't understand God's laws of health and healing. This well-known professor of computer engineering felt tired and jaundiced one day. His doctor finally diagnosed him with pancreatic cancer. They found a spot on his pancreas and said there was literally no hope. According to medical statistics, ninety-six percent of pancreatic cancer patients die within five years of diagnosis. He was told chemotherapy treatment would only prolong his life for a little while. The best cancer treatments usually don't extend people's lives longer than a few months, anyway.

Not long after Pausch was diagnosed with "incurable" pancreatic cancer in September 2006, treatment directives were given immediately. There would be the traditional oncological treatment of surgery and chemotherapy. Pausch was also told of the grim survival rates for patients with this type of cancer. Only one in five million live. Fifty percent are dead within six months. Eighty-four percent are expected to die within a year. And 96 percent are dead within five years. His belief system aligned with these medical statistics, and this became his reality. Was he aware that in medical schools those statistics are passed down verbatim in professors' lectures and textbooks influenced by the pharmaceutical/chemotherapy industry? They believe those statistics with religious-like conviction as though Moses delivered them from Mount Sinai. In addition, when these doctors begin to practice and see patients with pancreatic cancer, their perspective and belief system and thus their reality has already been molded and solidified. They know the statistics, have formed their view of reality, and they're legally and ethically bound to administer the mainstream cancer treatment. If perchance they decide to suggest an "alternative treatment," they could lose their license, face stiff penalties, fines, or a jail sentence.

Was hope given at all? Did Pausch ask the right questions? Is disease prognostication a self-fulfilling prophecy? Is there a psychosomatic effect when given a death sentence? How great is the effect of the mind on the body? Many medical statistics have shown that there is only a 10 percent genetic link to pancreatic cancer; which means that 90 percent of the time the disease's origin is environmentally linked or lifestyle induced. The website also clearly discusses that the majority of that 10 percent genetic link is more than likely expressed after birth, which also tells us that the disease is almost exclusively influenced by epigenetics or environment and lifestyle.

Deepak Chopra, endocrinologist, lecturer, celebrity and author of many books, states, "Prognostication is based on statistical probabilities. While statistics may apply to a large population sample, they tell us nothing about the individual. For example, if the average temperature in New York City for the year is 54 degrees Fahrenheit, that does not inform me what the temperature is today. Similarly, if you are a citizen of Bangladesh and the average income of a Bangladeshi is $65 per household per year, that does not tell me your income. When I was a medical student, there used to be a joke about statistics, which in today's climate of political correctness might be considered sexist, but at the risk of possibly offending some, I will share it with you anyway because it makes an insightful point. "Statistics are like a girl in a bikini. What she reveals is obvious, but what she conceals is much more interesting." As applied to illness, there is only one rule: Do not buy into the prognosis; you may be buying into a self-fulfilling prophecy.

Pausch's doctors doused his body with chemotherapy and he made the decision to accept the toxic poisons being poured into his body. Chemotherapy was developed during World War I. It was discovered that neurotoxins designed to kill soldiers could actually kill cancer in people's bodies. Like antibiotics, it's like dropping a nuclear bomb on a house to kill the mice. At any rate, Randy Pausch got this cancer treatment, assuming he was going to die, but hoping to buy more time. He went on the Oprah show and he started talking about his life, and he even received a seven-million-dollar contract to write a book. He started celebrating his life while preparing for his departure as he'd accepted the fact that he was going to die.

Again, there's a major flaw in that thinking and in that health model. The problem is that medical doctors went to medical school, and in their medical textbooks it said that pancreatic cancer kills. It's one of the most virulent forms of cancer. The medical professor teaches it, and the medical students hear it and adopt it as their belief system.

Through quantum physics, however, we know that reality is usually created by one's belief system. Quantum physics says an object can't be measured without the observer influencing what they're observing; so we know that intention and belief system determines a lot of what you're observing and so your belief system determines reality to a large extent. So if you or a loved one were given a terminal diagnosis and a doctor's belief system was that you're going to die, would you believe this or look for other answers?

Ultimately, this book is about hope. Do you know what I would have asked in Randy Pausch's case? I would have asked, "If 96 percent of people are dead in five years, but 4 percent are alive, what do I need to do to be in the 4 percent?" As a wellness doctor of the future, my new vision for America has people asking: "How do I not die from all the cancer and the heart disease and the strokes and all the things destroying Americans? What do I need to do to become part of that 4 percent?" If you are asking that question, you have hope. There is a way to live because, obviously, 4 percent are living.

Maybe Randy Pausch's doctors never asked the right questions: Is the nerve that's coming out of his back and going to his pancreas functioning properly? Is it being blocked or pinched? Is he getting the right nerve supply to his pancreas? Is there an atlas subluxation affecting his brain-stem region? Are the messages being blocked or interrupted? Is his brain stem delivering the right messages to the pancreas? Has his spine been checked? What about his diet? Has he been exposed to chemicals? Neurotoxins? Maybe he has mercury fillings in his teeth that are causing problems. Maybe he took toxic vaccines. Maybe he was getting the flu shot annually and the neurotoxic mercury in it poisoned his body, specifically his pancreas. Maybe he was under a lot of stress, drinking five pots of coffee a day, eating candy bars all day, and not putting the right foods in his body, causing chemical, physical, and emotional interference.

Pancreatic cancer is a lifestyle disease, not a genetic one, and no matter what anybody says, lifestyles can be changed. It has been proven scientifically that lifestyle changes can restore a person back to health and wholeness. Randy Pausch died on July 25, 2008. It wasn't his fault that he died. I believe in the end it was simply a matter of him not having access to a doctor who could show him how to make it to the 4 percent and how to get well from this primarily lifestyle-induced disease. It's not a terminal illness, and that's been proven. Please understand, I mean no dishonor to those who have died of pancreatic cancer or have lost a loved one. I only offer hope.

The principle of chiropractic is all about teaching the world how to be part of that 4 percent, not the 96 percent who may choose to believe in a statistical death sentence. As chiropractors, we stand in the gap, and shout to the world that yes, there is hope. Yes, you can live life without fear. Yes, the power that made the body can heal the body. Yes, God needs no help to heal, just no interference. The principled chiropractor empowers their patients to think within a new paradigm, thus enabling them to ask better questions and make more intelligent decisions. We understand that your thought process, more often than not, can be a matter of life and death.

> *"I desired to know why one person was ailing and his associate, eating at the same table, working in the same shop, at the same bench, was not. Why? What difference was there in the two persons that caused one to have pneumonia, catarrh, typhoid, cancer, or rheumatism, while his partner, similarly situated, escaped? Why?*
>
> *"D.D. Palmer, founder of the great profession of chiropractic The 1910 Chiropractor's Adjuster*

LEAVING A LEGACY

What we teach as wellness chiropractors is an understanding of the laws of health and healing. There's hope for you if you ask the right questions and make the right lifestyle changes. This is the message we strive to deliver to the next generation. This means making sure that your family has as little interference as possible. We live in an environment that is like a chemical soup. You're never going to remove all the interferences from your body because it's not a perfect world, but you can make sure that your family is growing up with as little interference to their neurological systems as possible.

RAISING UP THE NEXT GENERATION, BUILDING THE VISION

If we're going to focus on developing a strong healthy future nation, then we must start with our children. How do we go about raising and developing children who can function and perform at their best? One of the ways to accomplish this is to help them develop a titanium-like immune system. In order to achieve this, we need to first look at the chemicals with which we've traditionally subjected their bodies.

In 2009 the *American Journal of Pediatrics* released a statement that children and adults should not be taking "cold" medications. They have been shown to damage the body and the normal development of the immune system and can actually create disease. Phenylpropylalanine, an active ingredient, has been implicated in the cause of strokes, brain bleeding, and seizures. Thank God that this cold medicine fiasco was finally exposed after decades of harming children. Almost every common over-the-counter childhood cold and flu remedy has at one time contained phenylpropylalanine, "Cold medicines are useless," say pediatricians who petitioned the FDA to ban the marketing of such products to children. In 2008, an FDA advisory panel partially agreed with their recommendations, and voted to declare that such medicines should not be used in children younger than six. As far as I know, there has never been a single clinical trial proving these medicines to be either safe or effective for use in children.

Additional ways to raise up the next generation to be their best is to implement the following: Give them plenty of clean water and sea salts. Half their body weight in ounces is a good place to start. Add a green powder (i.e. Supergreens or Green Vibrance – see appendix for more information on these products) and lemon. This will help with cleansing and detoxification. As much as possible eliminate white sugar from their diet. Sugar is fertilizer for bacteria, viruses, yeast, mold, cancer, and diseases of all kinds. When Lauric acid is consumed in the diet either in human breast milk or in coconut oil, it forms a mono-gyceride called monolaurin, which has been shown to destroy several bacteria and viruses, including hysteria monocytogenes, helicobacter pylori, and protozoa such as giardia lamblia. Some of the viruses that have been destroyed by monolaurin include, measles, herpes simplex virus, influenza, and cytomegalovirus. There is also evidence now that the medium-chain triglycerides in coconut oil kill yeast infections such as candida.

Many doctors today also recommend letting children's symptoms express themselves naturally. Coughing, sneezing, sweating, headaches, stuffy noses, shivering, and diarrhea, among others, are all lifesaving mechanisms which aid in cleansing and detoxifying poisonous waste from their body. Many doctors are recommending letting the fever burn (unless the child becomes listless, lethargic, or unresponsive, in which case it's considered a medical emergency). At 102 and 103 degrees, interferon is released in large quantities. Interferon is the substance that strengthens the immune system and is arguably the most powerful cancer killer found in the body.

Also, most medical authorities agree that aspirin should not be given to a child or teenager who has a fever, especially if the child also has flu symptoms or chicken pox. Aspirin can cause a serious and sometimes fatal condition called Reye's syndrome in children. If you don't let the body fight on its own and let the immune system be challenged, the child will more than likely develop a weak, sick, and diseased immune system. The immune system must be challenged like a muscle; if not, it can become weak, sick, and diseased. A healthy, tough immune system is flexible, responsive, and strong, and when challenged by an invader it recovers quickly after winning each of its battles. Just as we've learned in earlier chapters that stress is vital for the healthy development and functioning of muscles, the same principle applies to our immune system. When animals are experientially raised in a germ-free environment from birth, their immune systems become severely underdeveloped compared to those of animals raised in normal conditions. As a result, the overly protected animals live only a short time outside their original germ-free environment before disease overwhelms their stunted immune systems.

"Sniffles, sneezes, and fever are good for you. They clear the airways of harmful irritants and allergy-causing substances. Fevers actually fight viral and bacterial infections. And diseases are shortened by letting the fever run its course. Coughing rids the body of bacteria and virus by way of the lungs. Taking fever-reducing drugs or cough suppressants can lead to pneumonia or more serious respiratory infection," states Dr. William B. Greenough, professor at Johns Hopkins School of Medicine. Parents, remember: Symptoms are the way the body heals itself and the way you develop children with powerful, strong bodies. This is the legacy that we can leave.

NEW VISION HEALING BASICS FOR CHILDREN

As you've learned thus far, the brain and spinal cord run, coordinate, control, harmonize, and govern every aspect of your health and your existence. God put the most amazing healing power in the brain and spinal cord. This power is what runs your body and heals your body. Without a proper functioning nerve system you cannot be well. For your child to be well, the brain must be able to communicate with the body and its organs through the spinal cord, which is housed by the spine. If you want your child to be well, you need to keep the nervous system well. If your child is "sick," or as we say at YFCC, "expressing health", then you absolutely need to get your child adjusted. In clinical trials, getting adjusted has been shown to possibly boost immunity up to 200 percent. Clinically, we see that in almost every case the main cause of a potentially "dangerous" fever is a damaged nerve system due to subluxation. A child's fever will not burn properly if there is interference to the system that controls the creation and regulation of fevers in the human body. Considering all the falls, accidents, and traumas that the typical child experiences, it stands to reason that so many children have subluxation that weakens their immune systems and in many cases possibly creates problems such as headaches, allergies, sinus issues, auditory problems, dizziness, motor problems, and other neurological disturbances.

"Drugs never cure disease. They merely hush the voice of nature's protest, and pull down the danger signals she erects along the pathway of transgression. Any poison taken into the system has to be reckoned with later on, even though it palliates present symptoms. Pain may disappear, but the patient is left in a worse condition, though unconscious of it at the time."
–Daniel. H. Kress, M.D.

THE VACCINE DILEMMA AND
YOUR CHILD'S FUTURE

In many scientific papers, vaccines have been linked to sickness, disease, and speculated in many cases of death. The children whom I see get vaccinated in a clinical setting develop a severely weakened immune system and often manifest disease shortly thereafter. The most common diseases that have been reported by patients of mine have been autism and learning disabilities. What you may not know is that the MMR [Measles, Mumps, Rubella] Vaccine and the Varicella [chickenpox] vaccines are both propagated [grown] on tissue derived from aborted babies. The cells are called "human diploid cells" in the product description. There's more bad news for advocates of the MMR (measles-mumps-rubella) vaccine with the discovery that it can cause a blood disorder. Researchers have found that it may trigger idiopathic thrombocytopenic purpura (ITP), an immune system malfunction that destroys the body's own blood platelets. "There has been a tenfold increase in autism and related forms of brain damage over the past fifteen years in England, roughly coinciding with MMR's introduction, and an extremely worrying increase in childhood inflammatory bowel diseases and immune disorders such as diabetes, and no one in authority will even admit it's happening, let alone try to investigate the causes," wrote Dr. S. Corrigan in the Daily Mail in 2007.

According to the current vaccine schedule, by six months of age, a child is to be injected with forty-eight vaccines. At eighteen months, the average toddler is to be injected with seventy vaccines and by the age of six is scheduled to endure eighty-nine vaccines, which is up from seventy-four in 2002.

"Between fifteen and twenty percent of American schoolchildren are considered learning disabled with minimal brain dysfunction directly caused by vaccine damage," According to H. L. Coulter, author of Vaccination, Social Violence and Criminality: The Medical Assault on the American Brain.

Even in populations that are fully vaccinated, outbreaks have occurred – and 80 percent of all cases of measles are contracted in vaccinated people, according to the Morbidity and Mortality Weekly Report.   In 1975 Japan raised the minimum age of vaccination from two months to two years. Crib death, infantile seizures, meningitis, and other infectious diseases in infants virtually disappeared. Japan went from seventeenth in infant survival in the world to number one.

What parents usually discover is that some, but not all pediatricians appear to act as vaccine salespeople as evidenced by the little they know about these products. Once parents are armed with the right knowledge and can ask the right questions, it is much easier for them to say "no" and seek health care elsewhere. Below is a list of questions to which parents need to get answers. They are as follows:

1. Are vaccinated children healthier than nonvaccinated children?

2. Do vaccines have any long-term side effects or damage that may not surface for months or years?

3. Does research show vaccines are safe?

4. Can vaccines cause cancer or fertility problems?

5. Do vaccines cause SIDS (Sudden Infant Death Syndrome, also known as crib death)?

6. What are the chances that my child may be hurt or killed by a vaccine?

7. Do the assumed benefits of vaccination outweigh the risks?

8. Didn't vaccines get rid of acute infectious childhood diseases?

9. What about polio? Wasn't it eliminated due to vaccination?

10. Was the polio shot given in the 1950s and '60s contaminated with monkey virus? Is it causing cancer?

11. Is vaccination why we have so much cancer today?

12. Are there benefits to a child having acute infectious childhood diseases?

13. Are the ingredients in vaccines safe?

14. How do vaccines work on a cellular level? How do vaccines affect the immune system/nervous system on a cellular level? How do vaccines cause damage on a cellular level?

15. Do vaccines affect genetic material? Are we hurting future generations?

16. Is there a conflict of interest in vaccine policy decisions?

17. Can a person legally avoid vaccinations?

If the above questions weren't thought-provoking enough, check out some of the common ingredients found in vaccines (note: not all are ever put into a single vaccine).

2 - Phenoxyethanol

2-(ethylmercurithio) benzoic acid

3-0 Desacyl-4 Monophosphoryl lipid

Acetic acid

Acid hydrolysate (casein)

African green monkey kidney cells

alcohol

alpha-tocopheryl

Aluminum

Aluminum adjuvant

Aluminum hydroxide

Aluminum hydroxyphosphate sulfate

Aluminum oxide

Aluminum phosphate

Aluminum potassium sulfate

Amino acids

Aminoglycoside (antibiotic)

Ammonium sulfate

Amphotericin B

Anhydrous disodium phosphate

Arum triphyllum

AS04C containing 3-O-desacyl-4-
monophosphoryl lipid

Ascorbic acid

Aspartame

Bacillus anthracis

Belladonna

Benzethonium chloride

Beta-propiolactone

Boric acid

Bovine (cow) serum

Calcium carbonate

Calcium chloride

Casamino acids (casein)

Cephalin (antibiotic)

Chick embryo cells

Chinese hamster ovary cells

Chlortetracycline hydrochloride

Cholera virus

Dehydrate sodium hydrogen phosphate

Dextran

Dextrose

Dibutyl phthalate

Diethyl phthalate

Diethylether

Diphtheria CRM197 protein

Diphtheria formoltoxoid

Diphtheria toxoid

Disodium dehydrogenate phosphate

Disodium edentate (EDTA)

Disodium phosphate dehydrate

Dog kidney cells

Dulbecco's Modified Eagle Medium

Egg protein

Erythromycin (antibiotic)

Ethylene glycol

Ethylenediaminetetraacetic acid (EDTA)

Fatty-acid ester-based antifoam

Ferrum phosphoricum

Fetuin

Filamentous hemagglutinin (FHA)

Formaldehyde

Formalin

Galactose

Gelatin

Gentamicin Sulfate

Glutamate

Glutaraldehyde

Glycerine

Glycine

Glycol p-isooctylphenyl ether

Haemophilus influenzae B

Hemagglutinin culture flu viruses of type A(H1N1), A(H3N2)

Hemin chloride

Hexadecyltrimethylammonium bromide

Histidine

HPV-16 L1 protein

HPV-18 L1 protein

Human albumin

Human cell line: PER C6

Human diploid cells (WI-38)

Human Diploid cells: MRC5 proteins

Hydrochloric acid

Hydrocortisone

Hydrogen succinate

Hydroxypropyl methycellulose phthalate

Influenza A virus hemagglutinin

Influenza B virus hemagglutinin

Influenzae polysaccharides

Iron oxide red ci77491

Iron oxide yellow ci77492

Isotonic phosphate buffered saline

Isotonic saline

Isotonic sodium chloride solution

Kanamycin (antibiotic)

L-alanine

L-histidine hydrochloride

Lactose

Latex

Lecithin

Lipoprotein OspA

Liquid light paraffin

M phosphate- buffered saline

Magnesium chloride hexahydrate

Magnesium stearate

Magnesium sulfate

Mannitol

Marcol 82 (R)

Medium 199

Meningococcal Group C oligosaccharide

Meningococcal group C polysaccharide

Meningococcal polysaccharide serogroup Y

Meningococcal polysaccharides W135

Mercurius solubilis

Mercury

Mertiolyat

MF59

Mineral oil

Mineral salts

Minimum Essential Medium

Monopotassium glutamate

Monopotassium phosphate

Monosodium Glutamate (MSG)

Monosodium phosphate

Montanide 80 (R)

Mouse brain cells

Neisseria meningitides OMPC

Neomycin

Neomycin sulphate

Nicotinamide adenine dinucleotide

Octoxynol-10

Ovalbumin (egg)

Pertactin

Pertussis toxin

Pertussis Toxoid

Phenol

Phospholipids lecithin

Pneumococcal Polysaccharide(s)

Polyalcohols

Polydimethylsiloxane

Polyethylene glycol

Polygeline

Polymyxin B

Polyoxidonium

Polyribosylribitol phosphate

Polysorbate 20

Polysorbate 80

Potassium chloride

Potassium dehydrogenate phosphate

Potassium dihydrogen phosphate

Potassium diphosphate

Potassium glutamate

Potassium monophosphate

Potassium phosphate

Potassium phosphate- monobasic

Protein contaminants

Protein hydrolysate

Rabies antigen

Rabies: Human Immunoglobulin Antibodies

Recombinant HBsAg protein

Saline solution

Salmonella Typhi bacteria

Silicon

Sodium acetate

Sodium bicarbonate

Sodium Borate

Sodium carbonate

Sodium chloride

Sodium citrate

Sodium deoxycholate

Sodium dihydrogen phosphate dehydrate

Sodium EDTA

Sodium hydrogen carbonate

Sodium hydroxide

Sodium phosphate

Sodium phosphate- dibasic anhydrous

Sodium phosphate-dibasic dodecahydrate

Sodium phosphate-monobasic

Sodium taurodeoxycholate

Sodium tetraborate decahydrate

Sorbitane mono-oleate

Sorbitol

Soy peptone

Soy protein

Squalene

Stopper vial may contain dry latex rubber

Streptomycin

Succinic Acid

Sucrose

Superficial glycoproteins
(gemagglutinin and neyroamynidasa)

Tetanus

Tetanus formoltoxoid

Tetanus protein

Tetanus toxin

Tetanus toxoid

Thimerosal

Titanium dioxide

Tri(n)butylphosphate

Triton N101

Triton X-100

Trometamol

Tryspin

Vibrio polysaccharide antigen

Virus: Coxiella burnetii organisms, killed

Virus: Hepatitis A

Virus: Hepatitis B

Virus: Human papillomavirus (denatured) (HPV)

Virus: Inactivated whole avian influenza

Virus: Influenza

Virus: Influenza virus antigens

Virus: Japanese encephalitis (JE)

Virus: Measles

Virus: Mumps

Virus: polio

Virus: Rabies

Virus: Respiratory Syncitial Virus (RSV)

Virus: Rotavirus (live, attenuated)

Virus: Rubella

Virus: SV40

Virus: Vaccinia (smallpox)

Virus: Varicella (chickenpox)

Virus: Yellow fever

Xanthan gum

Yeast

Yeast extract

KNOW THE TRUTH AND KNOW YOUR RIGHTS

For more information on vaccinations, check out the following resources:

1. WWW.NVIC.ORG

2. WWW.CHILDHOODSHOTS.COM

3. WWW.MERCOLA.COM

4. WWW.BRAINGUARDMD.COM

5. WWW.NOVACCINE.COM

6. WWW.VACLIB.ORG

7. WWW.ARI.ORG

8. WWW.VACCINESAFETY.EDU

9. WWW.CCID.ORG

10. WWW.VACCINETRUTH.COM

THE DANGERS OF ANTIBIOTIC USE
IN CHILDREN AND ADULTS:

Often times antibiotics are prescribed to children who are burning fevers or who are 'fighting colds'. It is important for parents to understand that antibiotic use early in life is thought, by some experts, to be linked to asthma, allergies, and many other diseases. My clinical experience has shown that in almost all cases a fever over 105 degrees is only dangerous when it's chemically induced. Clinically, I've seen that most uncontrollable fevers are created by a malfunction and weakening in the child's nerve system and immune system often caused by previous use of various medications including cold medications, vaccines, or antibiotics. As I have witnessed in a clinical setting, a fever will tend to burn abnormally when the child is subluxated as well.

The following quotes are the perspectives of many highly respected experts:

"Treating bacterial infections with antibiotics is like putting kerosene on an already burning fire"

-Dr. Robert O. Young

"Patients who did not take antibiotics had a higher rate of recovery than those who did; the rate of recovery did not differ between different types of antibiotic. Antibiotic treatment did not improve the rate of recovery of patients in this study."

-British Medical Journal, 1990

"The University of Washington found that if you filled twenty-five or more prescriptions for antibiotics over seventeen years, you doubled your risk of cancer."

-Time, Dec 6, 2004

"Infants exposed to one single round of antibiotics during their first year of life are twice as likely to develop asthma as those who don't. The more courses of antibiotics, the worse the immunity and the greater the risk of asthma."

—Newsday, March 6, 2006

"Antibiotics don't just lead to an increase in the risk of asthma. Antibiotics destroy our normal flora, which has severe adverse effects on the immune system function, digestion and absorption, and vitamin production. This adversely affects the function of every cell in the human ecosystem and significantly contributes to the development of illness. Deficiency in our normal flora also leads to the colonization of pathogenic flora, especially yeast and gram negative bacteria."

—Dr. James L. Chestnut of The Wellness Practice-Global Self Help Corp

"Researchers attempted to study how long the ill effects of antibiotics last by studying people for six months. At the end of six months, people still showed low resistance and poor immunity, leading the researchers to conclude that they have no idea how long-lasting or how damaging the effects of antibiotics truly are."

-The Clinical Advisor, April 2007

"The basic message is that treating a patient with an antibiotic will cause a dramatic change of his normal [bacterial] flora and select for resistant genes that can spread to a true pathogen (disease),"

- lead researcher Herman Goossens, M.D., Ph.D.,in a Lancet podcast interview.

"In our almost messianic quest to wipe out childhood disease through vaccinations, antibiotics and fever-reducing drugs – medical doctors have produced a wasteland of children who are literally chronically sick and tired, spending lives feeling uncomfortable in their untransformed skins. It is as if we have prevented caterpillars from becoming butterflies because the time of immobility as a chrysalis can be dangerous. Well it is dangerous, at least a little, but it is more dangerous—in fact deadly—to never allow a child to fulfill his or her destiny and become a butterfly. We urgently need to respect the transformative power of illness, to pluck up our courage and not succumb to those who promise better health through injecting us with poisons, or harsh anti-life medicines that become less and less effective. And more than anything we need to believe in the healing powers of our children's bodies, so we can give them the gift of confidence in their own strength as they embark on the challenges of adulthood."

—Thomas Cowan, M.D.

GIVING YOUR CHILD THE GIFT OF LIFE

Comparative studies of children raised under chiropractic wellness care vs. those raised under traditional allopathic care showed that chiropractic children were less prone to infections such as otitis media (inner ear infections) and tonsillitis, and that their immune systems were better able to cope with allergens than the medically raised children. The children raised under the chiropractic wellness model used fewer antibiotics and pharmaceuticals overall. They also recovered far faster from ear infections, allergies, colds, bouts of pneumonia, flu viruses, and injuries.

We are passionate about keeping children and babies healthy at YFCC. It is our mission to make sure the families of our community receive all the knowledge and resources necessary to live a life of health and vitality. Given that 65 percent of all neurological development occurs in the first year of life, having your baby checked early is of utmost importance. The nervous system is the system that interprets the environment. A child who does not properly receive information from the environment because of subluxation will have a distorted reality and diminished ability to express health. As a result of subluxation-induced neurological disruption, these children will grow up being less than they could be.

EXERCISE HELPS A CHILD

DEVELOP A BRIGHT MIND:

1. It stimulates formation of new, healthy brain cells.

2. It improves mental performance.

3. It enhances cognitive and memory performance.

4. It improves blood flow to the brain.

5. It improves attentional capacity, concentration, learning ability, and performance.

6. It enhances creative thinking, verbal skills, and decision-making.

7. It enhances growth hormone production.

8. It improves logical reasoning, recall, visual recognition, and speed of reaction.

9. It improves mood, alleviates depression, and improves quality of sleep.

MONKEY SEE, MONKEY DO!

It all starts with the parents. Parents need to start living this lifestyle if they want their children to live it. Children model, mimic, and pattern their lifestyle choices after the parents. If parents will stop monitoring symptoms and start monitoring function, they will take a huge step toward raising a healthy family. You have to have your nervous system evaluated including thermal readings, EMGs, and a nervous system checkup. That's the primary way to know if you're functioning well, not by symptom monitoring. I teach parents that they should not wait for the disease before they start doing something about it. It's not about early detection. It's all about prevention. Being proactive is the key.

The following are conditions that may exist, in adults and children, without overt signs or symptoms throughout their course, or without overt signs or symptoms until their end stages:

Arrhythmia	Hyperbilirubinemia
Atherosclerosis	Hypertension
Atriventricular block	Osteoarthritis
Benign prostatic Hypertrophy	Osteoporosis
Breast cancer	Ovarian cancer
Carcinoid syndrome	Ovarian cyst
Cardiomyopathy	Paget's disease
Cervix erosion	Pilonidal cyst
Cervical pondylosis	Polycystic kidney
Cervical cancer	Polycythemia
Colorectal cancer	Polyps of large bowel
Cholelithiasis	Prostate cancer
Coccidioidomycosis	Pyelonephritis
Cor pulmonale	Renal calculi
Coronary disease	Renal failure (chronic)
Diabetes mellitus	Retinoblastoma
Diverticular disease	Scoliosis
Emphysema	Tooth decay
Encephalitis	Tuberculosis
Fibroid tumors	Valvular heart disease
Glomerulonephritis	

I'd like to see this book and its ideas get into the school system. I want to see parents and teachers working together to make sure that students have a healthy, nontoxic environment in which to work and learn. My heart really is with the families, parents, teachers, and students. That's why I believe this information must get into the schools and get to the students, and we must begin creating these habits at the earliest age possible.

MY DRUG ADVICE

I am not a qualified drug expert and do not possess a medical/drug license. I am not a medical doctor, nor can I administer drugs or tell a patient to discontinue them, but I'll tell you from my own clinical experience what I've seen: All drugs should be avoided except the ones that are keeping people alive. I cannot give medical recommendations because it's illegal for me to do so, but I avoid medications at all costs, and with valid exceptions regarding removed or altered organs. Your wellness lifestyle should allow you to be able to avoid most, if not all, drugs, with the obvious exception of emergency or crisis care; which is unavoidable in urgent situations. Genuine health care focuses on quality of life, performance, and potential. This means that a person doesn't look at health care as fighting disease with drugs and a constant biochemical war being waged on the human body to kill invaders and "disease causing germs," but rather for the purposes of improving overall health and well-being and developing an extraordinary quality of life.

"DOCTOR, HEAL THY SELF"

A great doctor is, without question, someone who can produce results. These results are also produced and are demonstrated in the doctor's own life and family's life. I often have had patients whose general medical doctor or cardiologist told them to lose forty pounds, eat better, and start exercising. Ironically the doctor himself was eighty pounds overweight, smoked cigarettes, ate junk food, and didn't exercise a day in his life. The doctor you see should have a track record of producing results on a daily basis and who has examples of people you can speak with or read their written testimonials. The doctor you choose should be a loving, caring, compassionate man or woman who is expertly trained in removing the three interferences. They should not only be highly qualified and trained to deliver exceptional care, but they and their families should demonstrate that they live a wellness lifestyle. They walk their talk. They are a living, breathing, walking, talking picture of what a healthy lifestyle should look like. The best way to find good health management and coaching is by referral. Ask around your town and see who is recommended. Again, in my opinion, family wellness-oriented chiropractors produce the best results. They truly understand how the body gets sick and most importantly how to get people well and keep them well for the rest of their lives, with the best chance of eliminating the need for drugs and surgery.

I want you to know that no matter how badly you've hurt yourself, the body is extraordinarily forgiving. The body is wonderfully made, and God put amazing healing powers in it. Through a change in diet that supports a more alkaline system (which includes a large amount of good fats and green vegetables and minimal amounts of flour, grains, caffeine, sugar, and pasteurized dairy products), increased hydration, proper spinal alignment, posture restoration, and muscular balancing, you can overcome degenerative organ, joint, and muscle conditions. They are not a permanent sentence. It doesn't matter where you are in life, a newborn or ninety, these principles apply to you. There are unlimited possibilities for you and everyone you know, and the first step is applying the concepts and principles of this book.

Remember, health is a process, not an event. Your goal is progress, not perfection. You can set yourself up to be sick, or you can choose to be healthy and vibrant. The choice is always yours.

"Step-by-step: I can't think of any other way of accomplishing anything." -Michael Jordan (greatest basketball player to ever live)

CHAPTER NINE

TESTIMONIALS

"Show me your faith without deeds, and I will show you my faith by what I do. Since by keeping the body in health and vigor one walks in the ways of God. It being impossible during sickness to have any understanding or knowledge of the creator, it is a Man's duty to avoid whatever is injurious to the body, and to cultivate habits conducive to health and vigor."

—Moses Maimonedes, 12th-century Jewish scholar

Three times each year, our office conducts a life-transforming event that teaches everything from A-Z regarding health and wellness. I inform attendees that the information they acquire during the course of the program will allow them to develop an encyclopedic knowledge of health and wellness. And the program will certainly equip them with everything they need to live an ultimately healthy lifestyle. On the following pages, I've included personal testimonials from patients who've attended our one-day and six-week transformational events. They tell "before and after" stories in regards to their involvement with our events and programs as well as their experience as Yachter Family Chiropractic patients.

FROM CAROL COPELAND

Harry S. Truman once said, "It's what you learn after you know it all that counts." Well, I thought I had already learned all I needed to know from the past two Extreme Make-Overs that I attended but decided I would participate in this one to hear the new information that was being promoted. I learned more than I ever wanted to know and find it totally amazing that I'm still alive and in good health after fifty years of chemicals, mercury fillings, and processed foods. Ignorance is bliss, but now that I know better, I must make changes in my life if I want to live longer than my parents, who died at seventy and seventy-one. The past five weeks flew by, and I only just started customized nutrition changes in the fourth week. I think my brain was still trying to process all the information that it was absorbing. The Twinkie demonstration will stay in my memory forever! My body may not have changed in appearance the way I'd like it to, but it's the "stuff" that's not seen that has undergone a transformation. I have my carotid arteries checked every two years by ultrasound for my own peace of mind since I don't want to end up in a wheelchair from strokes like my twin brother. Anyway, two years ago they showed "mild" plaque build-up. The results of the ultrasound I took three weeks ago showed no plaque at all, so I know I'm going in the right direction. I intend to continue this lifestyle forever even though it's made me an outcast among friends and family who think I'm crazy. I do try my hardest to educate them so they'll understand why I do what I do (chiropractic adjustments, exercise, supplements, and proper nutrition).

Thanks so much to Dr. Dan and his staff for their outstanding dedication and passion for bringing the chiropractic lifestyle to this community.

FROM VALARIE ENTERS (A YFCC PATIENT)

Everyone who is born needs chiropractic care. It is a fundamental in life. Why? Because human beings are active; and in that activity our bones are apt to shift and change. Sometimes it's because of the stressors we face; sometimes it's from the birth process itself. And of course, because of various accidents that occur. My entire family (including three children) has reaped great benefits from consistent chiropractic adjustments.

I think what America has only seen is people popping pills in order to get rid of pain. There never really has been the presentation about chiropractic to the mass media that shows it's a viable option that has enjoyed great success. I know people who have witnessed my life know I don't get sick and know that I get regular chiropractic care. In two and half years at my job, I have never once called in sick. I know that chiropractic care is viewed as thinking outside of the box. It's not covered in my health insurance plan. I have to pay outside of that. When people ask me about that, I tell them, "Listen, you are going to pay one way or another. Either pay ahead and be proactive, or pay through missed work, school, prescriptions, or missed life!" I'll pay ahead and keep enjoying life. Someday I hope America gets its act together and acknowledges chiropractic. But, I'm certainly not going to hold my breath. I do have health insurance, and that's for major medical emergencies. But I am more than willing to sacrifice some niceties in life to have chiropractic in it.

Our son Jack was born on February 10th, 1999. He was born with several challenges including subglottic stenosis, severe reflux, and swallowing issues that impaired his ability to eat. He had gross motor and fine motor issues and was unable to crawl until he was one year old, and he didn't walk until he was two. He could not eat by his mouth until he was three and a half, and then it was only very small amounts. He has a long list of doctors who tried to use traditional medicine to treat him. None of which brought true success. Jack has had a general pediatrician, pulmonologist, neurologist, gastroenterologist, otolaryngologist, early interventionist, physical therapist, occupational therapist, oral therapist, in-home nurse, and two eager parents! He was exposed to several drugs, therapies, and treatments. None of which healed him and some of which have left permanent damage on his body including hearing loss due to nerve damage from breathing treatments. Nothing we did through traditional medicine improved his life. We were told point blank that there were no surgeries that could be performed to rectify Jack's issues. And they were right. All those treatments may have only sustained his life. Jack had received the "best" that health care had to offer. At one point I considered the doctors, nurses, and therapists to be my only friends. After all, I spent more time with them and driving Jack to appointments than anywhere else! But with all the care Jack received, he still was unable to eat enough to sustain himself. We nearly had an open account at Walgreen's Pharmacy in order to supply all of Jack's medications. And these weren't cheap either! Jack's antibiotics were the same ones usually reserved for AIDS patients. The doctor explained to me that aggressive treatment was necessary in order to ward off any chance of pneumonia. No one ever mentioned chiropractors, or that regular adjustments boost the immune system. It wasn't until he received regular chiropractic adjustments that within one year's time, we witnessed Jack come off his feeding tube and flourish into a normal healthy young boy. He's been able to discontinue all his breathing treatment medicines, and his swallowing ability has greatly improved. He is eating exclusively by mouth, and his feeding tube has now been perma-

nently removed. His nervous system was the center of his issues. The doctors said that there was nothing they could do to help him. How right they were! Jack's issues were neurological, and the heart of his problem was with his brain. When his spine was aligned, his brain could channel the necessary power to his body. It was at the corpus collossum, or the white matter of his brain. Waking up the nervous system and stimulating it through regular adjustments gave Jack a new lease on life and set him on the path of success.

In the initial consult, Dr. Dan was clear that he would not promise to "heal" anyone. He did promise to remove interference and thus allow the central nervous system to flow freely through the spine. Dr. Dan said that only God could heal, and I firmly believed that He could use Dr. Dan to help Jack in his fight to eat by mouth.

Just recently we witnessed another everyday miracle of chiropractic. Jack had a fever and was eager to get back to his regular routine. I encouraged him to rest and let the fever do the work. Without using acetaminophen and within just a few hours, he was up and around and fever free!

If I could, I would ask the skeptics or individuals/families who have had previous negative experience with chiropractic what type of chiropractic care were they under. I would also talk to them about their lifestyle and their choices. Some people generally make bad choices in many areas in their life and would love to place the blame on something or someone. A life with chiropractic that focuses on God healing your body from the inside out, lotion and potion free, is a life of accountability. Right choices in nutrition and lifestyle will directly affect the results that chiropractic care has on life. You don't have to be a health freak or eat only soy to be whole and healthy. But the choices you make overall have a direct correlation as to what type of results you may experience. For me, being a part of chiropractic care is being part of a great community of people who understand that chiropractic is the foundation to building a healthy life. A skeptic would only need to see the results in my family's life. My son can now eat through his mouth, my family has lived without antibiotics for six years, my husband has had only a couple bad backaches in four years, and my backaches and stiff neck are gone. My sister got pregnant after twenty years of infertility. My mother-in-law was able to come off of numerous drugs and is healthier than ever! My sister-in-law had hearing restored in one ear after one chiropractic adjustment!

With chiropractic as a part of our everyday life, if and when we do feel something coming on, i.e. cold or flu, it's usually worked out of our system within a few days and I really never experience those sicknesses like I did before chiropractic. I think that it is because of the continued care I have received. It has built up my immune system and has woken up the perfect plan that was already in place in my body to do its job.

People need to know the main problem with medicine is that it is being used as a money-making machine instead of a method to help hurting people. The medical profession certainly has its place. It should be used to help people in medical emergencies.

Just realize that regarding the pharmaceutical companies, you are not seen as a person, you are seen as an opportunity to make money. Just look at the pattern of a drug. First everyone is excited about its prospects, some receive great results, there is a big splash, flashy ad in magazines and on TV then, hey, maybe it's not so great, and now didn't so-and-so die from it, and then come the lawsuits. NO THANKS!

The big train of health care is chugging along on its track to a destination that can never be reached. It's there for a purpose:

emergency medicine. I don't think that it will be long before the tide of "health" care changes. I have heard it called "crash" care. And that seems to be a more suitable name. I think that it would behoove people to create health-care savings accounts to rely on financially instead of participating in traditional health insurance.

The most important regimen to keep a family healthy is to make regular chiropractic adjustments a part of your life. Eating healthy is important; no need to be fanatical, but a healthy balance is important.   If you fail to get regular adjustments, you cannot expect to enjoy the results of them. If you start getting a cold, you can count that as a reminder to get yourself in the office and get an adjustment.

. Families need to share what they have experienced themselves. There should be classes throughout the community to educate those who have never known chiropractic in the way I have.

Here are additional life-changing events that have taken place in my extended family:

1. My mother-in-law Marion Enters went to Dr. Christian, a wellness chiropractor, and at the time was exhausted and on a variety of medications. She was able to come off most of her meds and is living an energetic life!

2. My sister-in-law Bonni Morrison is Dr. Christian's patient as well, and had her hearing restored after her sinus passages were cleared from an adjustment.

3. My friend Kathleen had migraine headaches and after adjustments was pain free. She was so moved, she cried.

4. My nephew said that he didn't want to be like his crazy cousins always getting adjusted, but now he is telling everyone how great chiropractic is!

5. *My sister Margaret could not conceive and after the initial chiropractic adjustments conceived and is expecting her first child!*

A FAMILY'S HEALING RESULTS AT
YFCC: A NOTE OF THANKS

Dear Dr. Dan,

It was December 2001 when we began seeing you. Hannah was five months and Emma had just turned three. This is when I woke up one morning with pain in all of my joints and swelling all over my body. I went to the emergency room and the doctor ran tests, which I didn't even know what he was checking for, and he told me that all of the tests came back negative, but we wouldn't know about the rheumatoid arthritis for a few days. He advised me to see a rheumatologist. The rheumatologist I saw ran his own tests and told me that my blood work was perfect, probably better than his own blood except that my ANA levels were off the charts; they were 1:1280 and they should be 1:45 or 1:70 (or something like that). When I asked for an explanation as to what is ANA, he said that it was too difficult to explain but that it indicates an autoimmune disease. He guessed that I probably had RH or Lupus or Scleroderma or maybe all of the above. He said that he couldn't specifically diagnose me because none of my internal organs had been affected. When I asked what I should do, he said that there was nothing to do; these things are chronic and degenerative and when one or more of my internal organs are affected, then he could make a diagnosis.

You may remember that when I told you this you told me to be careful as to what I accepted as truth and advised me to see you three times a week for adjustments and change my diet to no dairy, red meat, sugar, wheat and to exercise; which I began to do even as exhausted as I was with a new baby and a toddler. It took awhile, about two to two and a half years, and then I visited another rheumatologist (I fired the first one) and my blood tests came back with normal levels of ANA, 1:60. I began to cheer in the office and almost jumped up and down and I would have hugged the guy, but he sat motionless and emotionless and said, "Sometimes these things can fluctuate. I am going to refer you to the Mayo Clinic." Unbelievable!

I know that I didn't need to go to the Mayo Clinic, but just to prove a point, I did. The doctor there mocked the tests that showed 1:1280 for two years and then about four months after the last high ANA, there was the one test that showed 1:60. I said, "But there are two more tests spanning about eight months showing normal ANA." He scoffed again and said, "We'll do our own tests." He did and guess what, they were also normal. He decided to diagnose me with scleroderma anyway and said that I must be in the two percent with auto immune and normal ANA. He decided on the scleroderma because I have Raynaud's Phenomena and because he found that my esophagus is not moving the food down the way it should. When I asked what this means for me (I wondered exactly what would he be waiting for), he said that one day I may be eating and I may swallow and the food will get stuck and will not be able to go either way and then I would have to go to the ER and they would have to widen the esophagus and then it could possibly happen again at a later date. Then he prescribed one of the drugs for acid reflux. I said that I don't like to take drugs, and asked for an alternative. He said that there was no alternative. I also told him that I disagreed with his diagnosis.

I no longer have a need to see any rheumatologist. Initially, he accepted the diagnosis from the Mayo Clinic doctor, but now he disregards it and feels it was misdiagnosed! The really good news is that my little girls are healthy! I don't even remember the last time I took them to the pediatrician. I remember one time, a while ago, I brought Emma, I think for a check up. I had to pay ten dollars for them to get her records out of archives--sounds like a hoax to me. Emma rides horses and every now and then she takes a fall but since we see you regularly, I don't worry about it.

Thank you,

Mary Dipodova

MULTIPLE SCLEROSIS SYMPTOMS DISAPPEAR UNDER CHIROPRACTIC CARE

Below is a description of Phyllis' journey before and after coming to Yachter Family Chiropractic Center

What treatments did you try first? When diagnosed with multiple sclerosis, the medical doctors put me on steroids, then nothing for two years, then injections once a month.

What has principled chiropractic done for you? I can now wash my hair in warm or hot water and it doesn't make me sick. I can stand up and put on a pair of pants without falling over. I can take a shower without holding on to the shower wall. I can lie on my back on the floor and stretch out straight without having to put my feet up on a chair. I have a lot more stamina and energy. I wake up in the morning ready to get up instead of wanting to go back to sleep. I couldn't do these activities for the twelve years before I saw Dr. Dan. My legs have got that weightless feeling again. Before I saw Dr. Dan, every step I took felt like I was picking up fifty pounds with each foot. The dexterity in my fingers was gone; it is now back. This is the first thing I've written in twelve years (this was originally written down prior to typing it out). Also, if I tried to look at something on the side of the road, my truck would end up steering in that direction.

When I started seeing Dr. Dan I had hoped that it would stop some of the things, but I never imagined that it would stop all of it. It has! Thank you Dr. Dan Yachter.

Signed: Phyllis Kicklighter (she has been free of multiple sclerosis symptoms for over two years; complete recovery)

QUALITY OF LIFE RESTORED

From Dr. Dan's father, Sid Yachter:

It was the third time in my life that a watershed event was to happen. And for the third time it was chiropractically life-changing!

The first time:

I was about seven years old and away at summer camp. We were swimming in this beautiful lake that had a sliding pine sticking out in the middle of it. Apparently, I was the only one who didn't know there was a round metal tub sunk beneath the end of the slide with a fairly sharp lip on its perimeter. Head first I slid down, and ostensibly cracked open my skull on impact. A hair-line fractured skull and thirty stitches later, the camp doctor couldn't understand how I survived. For thirty some odd years afterwards, I would suffer from headaches, sometimes on a daily basis, sometimes from migraines, but always debilitating to various degrees.

Dr. David Yachter, my oldest son, was in his first term at Life Chiropractic College. At home, during his first semester break, he asked if he could try an adjustment that might help my chronic headaches. It only took a few seconds, but the occipital lift, which substantially moved my head off its atlas, gave me a rush and then a wonderful calmness. It had been subluxated all those years. Over time, whenever David came home from school, I'd get another adjustment, and gradually the headaches would disappear. I no longer have headaches. It was chiropractically life-changing.

The second time:

April 2001: It was a bike accident. Riding my twelve-speed around the development where I live, for whatever reason, at about 20 miles per hour I wound up flying over the handlebars. I landed squarely on my head, and with the exception of my jaw, most of my facial bones were shattered. By all accounts my neck and spinal column should have broken as well. But they did not. The only explanation was that for ten years I had been receiving chiropractic adjustment almost on a weekly basis. As a result, my neck and spinal column were supple enough to absorb the enormous impact. It took six months after major surgery, but I healed. I have almost no residual effects. It was chiropractically life-changing.

The third time:

Almost twelve years ago, my blood tests showed some serious problems. My triglycerides were 381, cholesterol at 275, and weight about 230 pounds. For me, these numbers were very dangerous, to say the least. Interestingly, I had no reaction nor response from the medical doctor who called for the blood work, not even a phone call. About six months ago, I again had a blood work-up. This time my triglycerides showed 263, Cholesterol at 168, and weight of 225 pounds. A little better, or so I thought. I sent these numbers to my younger son, Dr. Daniel Yachter, which sent shivers down his spine. He immediately called and we spoke for an hour and a half, discussing their significance and implications. Stressing the fact that I was a prime candidate for a heart attack, or even worse, a stroke, Daniel pushed hard for me to go on a "healing" diet. I was ready and took his advice to heart. Three months after I began the Healing Diet, I again had a blood work-up. The numbers showed that, with no medication, the Healing Diet works and works well. In addition to my triglycerides dropping to 57, HDL to 87, LDL to 101, my weight dropped by a totally unexpected 25 pounds (and by 35 pounds as of the publishing of this book). The rest of my vitals were well within the normal range. But that isn't the best part. After the first three months of dieting, I stopped using Prilosec (heartburn medication), and as of this writing I have been off Synthroid (thyroid medication) for a year. For the first time in 34 years, I am completely drug free! I am still on the Healing Diet, and it, too, has been a chiropractically life-changing experience for me!

PS. Daniel now says that at 68, I am starting to grow younger. If, by radically changing one's diet and receiving regular chiropractic adjustments so that all new drug-free healthy regeneration takes place on a cellular level, I believe my son the chiropractor has found the fountain of youth!

Sid Yachter

Every week, several more patients are liberated from their chemical shackles and medical prisons. Every day, lives are being transformed. Patients who once believed that they would have their illness, disease, or pain for life, and would never be able to stop medications, are now living in total health and vitality. These patients are now living a life without fear. These patients have broken out of their mental and physical chains and have begun to soar to heights never seen before. Below are two recent clinical cases.

PATIENT #1

Bryant Maulkey, age forty, taking eighteen medications at the same time, started care at YFCC on June 7, 2008. His doctors weren't sure if he had Type 1 or 2 diabetes, so they put him on medication for both.

Medical conditions:

- Type-1 and 2 diabetes
- High blood pressure
- Glaucoma
- Peripheral neuropathy
- Acid reflux
- High cholesterol
- Anaphalaxis to bee stings
- Protein in urine (kidney problems)

Medication list:

Apidra – 50 units three times/day for type-1 diabetes

Lantus – 80 units twice/day

Metformin – 1000 mg, one pill twice/day for diabetes

Lisinopril – 40 mg, one daily for blood pressure

Vytorin – 10-80 mg, once/day for cholesterol

Lyrica – 75 mg, twice/day for peripheral neuropathy

Cymbalta – 30 mg, once/day for peripheral neuropathy

Nexium – 40 mg, once/day for hiatal hernia and acid reflux

Mirapex – 0.5 mg, one at bedtime for restless leg syndrome

Slo-Niacin – 500 mg, one pill at bedtime (Niacin Antihiperlipidemic)

EpiPen – 0.3 mg, epinephrine auto injector as needed

AndroGel (testosterone gel) 1% pump – two pumps each/day

Betimol 0.5% ---three drops in both eyes twice/day for glaucoma

Trusopt 2% – one drop three times/day for glaucoma

Travatan (travoprost ophthalmic solution) .004% – one drop at bedtime.

Simvastatin – 40 mg, one tablet at bedtime for blood pressure

Hydrochlorothiazide – 25 mg, one tablet in morning for blood pressure

Aspirin – 85 mg, once/day for heart)

Progress Report:

Two weeks ago Bryant was able to stop taking all eighteen medications and is now living a drug-free life. No longer a diabetic, he has lost eighty pounds, and is no longer spending $5,600/month on medications. He says he feels better than ever. He didn't think he could feel so good! His subluxations/nerve interference are being corrected, and he is achieving a level of health never before imagined.

PATIENT # 2

Tony, age 49, started care at YFCC on June 16, 2008.

Medical conditions:

- High blood pressure

- Erectile dysfunction

- High pulse rate

- Vasovagal Syndrome

Medication list:

Heart medication

Cialis

Progress Report

In Tony's own words: "One month ago, I was weighing 290 pounds. After twelve adjustments and changes in my eating habits and diet (not eating after six o'clock in the evening, eating organic foods, drinking Udo's Oil and Supergreens, and cooking with coconut oil, my weight is 245 pounds. I had high blood pressure and an average pulse rate of seventy-five beats per minute or higher. My blood pressure was 140/95. My blood pressure after my first adjustment dropped to 107/65 and has stayed there for the last four weeks. After four weeks of chiropractic care, my pulse rate is also averaging fifty-five beats per minute. I was suffering from a condition called Vasovagal Syndrome, which is: a lack of coordination between the heart and the brain that in certain situations would cause a drop in tension, which would create a major deficiency in the amount of blood circulating to my brain. After the first adjustment, this condition was gone. I had erectile dysfunction, but after the first adjustment, it was gone. I went to three of the latest workshops at YFCC and listened and learned enough to start making the necessary changes to transform my lifestyle. I thank God for the opportunity of meeting Dr. Dan."

To watch and listen to these patients tell their stories, go to

YACHTERHEALTH.COM.

AND CLICK ON TESTIMONIALS.

HEALTHIER FAMILIES

The following testimonials come from YFCC patients who were compelled to share their personal stories of triumph.

Hi, friends and family!

This is long overdue, but something I feel led to share. Our family has recently celebrated a huge milestone. May 2008 was our year anniversary under chiropractic care. A year ago, we never thought it would be a date we would celebrate, but this journey definitely deserves a celebration. I just wanted to share a little about the past year for those of you who may not know much about it. For those of you who hear it over and over again, bear with me.

Over a year ago, our family was struggling with illness after illness. I was at my wit's end with giving my children prescription medications, and days or weeks later visiting the pediatrician's office yet again. Our

boys never had just a cold. It always started with a cold that led to an ear infection or turned into a respiratory infection. Both of our boys were diagnosed with RSV, and Kendall was even hospitalized for it. We were told they would both most likely end up with asthma and would probably be on breathing treatments during the entire "sick season." I was never OK with this information, but honestly didn't know any other way. With every illness, I would fight the feelings of knowing in my heart of hearts there was something else out there; there had to be! I could not imagine that this was the way God intended our children to start their precious lives. At one point, one or the other of our boys was sick for five weeks straight. Finally, one day I had a dear friend over when Kendall, my oldest, woke up with severe pain in his ear. I immediately did as I always did, and called to set up an appointment with our pediatrician. My friend asked some questions about Kendall's ears and then told me about their family chiropractor, Dr. Dan. She told me that he treats their whole family and teaches them about whole health and wellness, not just relieving pain in the neck and back. I called his office to inquire about setting an appointment and the following Monday was their Patient Appreciation Day.

During this year of treatment, we have learned amazing things about our bodies and about our children's health. I am so thrilled and blessed to report that our boys have not had a sick visit to the pediatrician since we have been under Dr. Dan's care. They have also been over a year without any medications of any kind (We were spending outrageous amounts of money on prescriptions and doctor visits). We are so excited and giving God the glory for that. We have had our share of colds and such, but our bodies are healthier and we are able to fight them off quickly. We literally don't get sick that often. We have noticed that when our boys do get sick, it is never to the extent it was before. It is truly a miracle, and I can't help sharing this information with others. If you would like to hear more about our story or would like more information on chiropractic care, please let me know. Thanks for taking the time to share in our journey.

Lots of love,

Heidi Lott

"I BELIEVE THAT THE EXTREME MAKEOVER IS SAVING MY LIFE."

I was introduced to Dr. Dan through a friend who invited me to the clinic when it was having a class to educate the community on molds and toxins. As a Realtor, I am always in and out of musty vacant homes and thought I might pick up a few tips on keeping myself safe. Little did I know that I was to receive a complete exam and full follow-up. I hadn't mentioned anything about past medical history, but it spoke for itself on the X-rays and nerve scans. I didn't have to say anything about my daily morning headaches or my L5-S1 ruptured disc that has been a problem from all those years ago. My headaches stopped immediately with my first adjustment.

I started my visits with Dr. Dan about the same time that we started the Extreme Makeover. I had already decided to dive into the makeover wholeheartedly. I've been working with a trainer for the past eleven months. I was happy with the weight loss and gain in lean muscle, but my weight loss hit a plateau about four months ago, and nothing changed that darn scale. I did as Dr. Dan suggested, removed all sugar and added coconut oil to my diet. In the first two weeks I lost three pounds. Not a lot, but it cemented my belief in the Healing Diet.

Now the big stuff – I contracted viral meningitis fifteen years ago. Believe it or not, it took the doctors months to come up with a diagnosis. First diagnosis was stroke, as I lost all my speech, short-term memory, and fine movements. (I could no longer write.) I also suffered full face paralysis, could barely walk, and had a horrible headache that took about six months to go away. Then they thought it might be multiple sclerosis before they finally decided on viral meningitis. I was given the strongest anti-viral medication available at the time. These were the same drugs given to AIDS patients. The doctors' greatest worry was that they were destroying my liver. Believe it or not, I was prescribed these anti-viral drugs for about five years. I have suffered many long-lasting effects from the virus's damage. There was the inability to sleep, loss of feeling in the bladder, loss of gag reflex, severe anxiousness, and the feeling that the volcano that lived inside my chest would blow up at any time. Naturally, the doctors prescribed their favorite medicine at the time, Paxil. I have been taking this poison for fourteen years. When I tried to withdraw, the side effects seemed to be worse than the poison. That is until Dr. Dan came along with his wonderful "Extreme Makeover." Like I said before, I jumped into this with both feet. Not only did I start the healing food diet, but I also stopped taking the Paxil. Yes, I am having some of the withdrawal symptoms that I previously suffered, but I am not getting the debilitating headaches that always happen with withdrawal from this medication. I believe that the Extreme Makeover is saving my life. I am now eating good healthy foods. I have increased the good fat in my diet and see Dr. Dan regularly.

Believe it or not, I contracted the viral meningitis while working in the operating room as a certified surgical technologist. I was the person standing across from the surgeons assisting them while they were performing surgery. Needless to say, after ten years working in the operating room, I am now as far away from that profession as I can get. Never did the doctors ever look at my diet or try to help in any way other than with pharmaceuticals. When you listen to Dr. Dan, getting and keeping yourself healthy sounds so obvious and easy to do. Why couldn't I have heard this fifteen years ago and saved myself from the misery and poisoning?

Thank you, Dr. Dan, for all that you do,

Signed,

A Very Happy YFCC Patient

AN AGGRESSIVE DEADLY CANCER GONE: ANOTHER HEALING AT YACHTER FAMILY CHIROPRACTIC CENTER

Clinical case

Mike Moton entered Yachter Family Chiropractic Center on Oct. 14, 2008. He began receiving chiropractic care and started the Extreme Makeover forty-day challenge shortly thereafter. Prior to entering YFCC, Mike's medical doctors had administered two sessions of chemotherapy in an attempt to destroy a rare form of deadly cancer known as pancreatic adenocarcinoma. The doctors gave him four to six months to live. After the second treatment, Mike decided to walk away from the chemotherapy and adopt a natural healing path, which included primarily chiropractic adjustments and healthy lifestyle changes such as an improved diet in which he ingested only organic meats, vegetables, and alkaline fruits. He became vigilant at food label reading and exercising, and he also enrolled in the YFCC detoxification program. Ninety days later, Mike's cancer is gone. He is healed!

What created Mike's extraordinary success? He followed everything we taught him at YFCC to the letter. He was an exemplary student, fully committed and engaged in the program, and he put his full trust in the power that made the body to heal the body. The doctors, of course, can't explain it.

To watch Mike tell his story, go to:

YACHTERHEALTH.COM,
CLICK ON THE TESTIMONIALS TAB

Here are other success stories of individuals and families who have completed our six-week transformational event

- Ellen has lost over ten pounds and no longer suffers from sleep apnea; her varicose veins have disappeared; and she is walking over three miles every weekend at our run/walk club. She was formerly clinically obese but has been set free from that prison.

- James Lawson at 78 years young has lost fifty pounds. No longer diabetic or taking medications, he is also off his heart medication, and off a total of ten other medications. He is more energetic and vital than he has been in over fifty years.

- Scott, Julie, Daniel, and Esther have experienced significant weight loss, dietary changes, major muscle mass improvements, and have experienced rapid nerve system correction. Scott notes, "I almost died today because of you! I went to workout this morning and decided that afterwards I would spend ten minutes in the sauna. Whenever I am in there I always talk to the other guys and share the success in my health thanks to Dr. Dan. Today they were so interested they kept asking questions, and when I would finish with one, another would walk in who they knew, and they would say, "Hey, Frankie, you have to hear this guy. And forty minutes later I stagger out of the steam room half dead. So if people come into the office but don't know the name of the guy who referred them, it was me. After showering, I heard one guy telling another: "You have to go see this guy; I will go with you."

- Ed and Nancy lost inches and pounds. Nancy went from a size 8 to size 4 dress. She is more energetic, sleeping better, and feels younger than ever. Ed has lost 70 pounds. Down from pant size 46 to 34. He works out at the gym daily and stopped smoking cigarettes. Pain in his neck and head are gone after twenty years, and he has more energy than he knows what to do with. He is also off all pharmaceuticals. They have attended every Extreme Makeover session as well.

YOUR DATE WITH YOUR SPECTACULAR DESTINY!

The Extreme Makeover one-day events and six-week events are held several times each year.
Please visit WWW.YACHTERHEALTHSOLUTIONS.COM
to register and begin the transformation!

Don't be left out!

1. Are you ready to maximize your life and your health?

2. Do you believe that God wants so much more for you?

3. Do you believe he has plans to help you prosper?

4. Are you ready to raise the bar?

5. Do you want to learn the secrets to incredible energy and vitality?

This is not a weight loss program – although if you attend the program, you'll learn how to lose all the weight you'd ever want to lose.

THE EXTREME MAKEOVER IS A LIFE-TRANSFORMATION PROGRAM!

Things you'll learn at the Extreme Makeover:

- The #1 cause of dis-ease

- How to increase your energy by at least 200 percent

- How to eliminate pain

- Drugless health strategies

- How to have outrageous health

- How to experience incredible happiness

- How to avoid getting the major disease killers in the U.S.

- How to reduce your risk of developing heart disease, stroke, cancer, diabetes, Alzheimer's disease, high cholesterol, high blood pressure, etc.

- How to extend your life

- Anti-aging strategies

- Detoxification/cellular cleansing strategies

- Customized nutrition and what diet is right for you

- Hormone balancing strategies to help you feel great

- God's eating principles

- Time and stress management

- Weight-loss strategies for rapid fat loss

- How environmental toxins can affect weight loss

- Exercise strategies that promote weight loss, not hinder it

- Burst training and four-minute workouts

- Making and tasting healthy foods

TAKE THE BULL BY THE HORNS AND ATTEND THE EXTREME MAKEOVER!

...A few more Extreme Makeover testimonials

"I would like to start out by first saying a big thank you to you and your whole staff, Dr. Dan, for presenting this powerful health information to the public. We are all misled so often by mass marketing. It was so good to hear the truth about how our body really works for us. This course was a lot to take in, but the basics are simple. Keep your system flushing and keep adding good stuff. As for my personal results, I am very pleased. The adjustments have allowed me to begin exercising regularly, something I could not do without a lot of pain before. I feel like you have helped me turn back the clock twenty years. Since the Extreme Makeover, in five weeks, I have lost eight pounds, my body fat has gone from 23 to 18 percent, and my BMI (body mass index) has dropped from 28 to 25 and I feel good. My light is brighter thanks to your teachings, Dr. Dan, and I look forward to the journey ahead.

Thanks again.

God bless, Jim V.

"I am especially grateful for the Extreme Makeover Workshop I attended, which included six weeks of intense training regarding nutrition, exercise, and life-changing goals. I have been enlightened to a healthful way of living. I have since made some lifestyle changes, especially in my diet. The use of the phytonutrient-rich foods has proved extremely helpful. My bowels function normally, and surprisingly my once

problematic acid reflux is practically gone. I am constantly encouraged to hydrate the system with the use of my pink one-liter polycarbonate bottle. I have also, along with the rest of my family, cut back on the intake of sweets, which has been difficult considering my sweet tooth. We have exchanged our use of vegetable oil for olive oil. My daughter is benefiting from burst training, which she incorporates into her daily exercise regimen. On a whole, Dr. Dan's teaching has raised our level of awareness. I now read labels while I grocery shop. If ingredients such as high fructose syrup, corn syrup, and hydrogenated fats are present, I remind myself that my family doesn't need it. I especially love YFCC's motto, "We move the bones, and God does the healing."

Thank you,

Jean James

YFCC testimonial:

As I near the completion of yet another Extreme Makeover, it's time to reflect on where I started, where I am now, and where I want to be in the future. Well, it all started back on a November afternoon in 1956. I was born a twin weighing 2 pounds, 3 ounces And given less than an hour to live. Oh, that's too far back!

I will backtrack five years to the point in my life where I had my gall bladder removed and, four months later, my thyroid. At 47, I felt like I was old and spent much of the next year trying to figure out how to change my life. Fortunately, I found Dr. Dan and YFCC. Almost immediately, my migraine headaches stopped and other various ailments gradually disappeared. I never missed my adjustments and did my exercises, but something was still missing. When I signed up for my first Extreme Makeover, I realized what it was. It was time to take control of my life even more and learn all I could. That's why I keep attending these events so that I can educate myself to live a longer life than my parents – Mom died at 71 and Dad, 11 months later, at 70 years old. I also don't want to end up in an Assisted Living Facility like my twin brother or take medications like my sister. Attending these Extreme Makeovers are my lifeline.

This particular EMO has been the most enjoyable, and when you participate and have fun, you retain more of the life-saving information that's given out each week. At the beginning of the EMO, I weighed in at 174 pounds, which was bad enough, but the real shocker was my body fat percentage. I was 43.8 percent fat, and my BMI showed I was obese. This was totally not acceptable. It's amazing how your eyes get opened when you see the numbers on paper. How did let myself get like this again? I knew I had to put in the time to really do it right, and permanently this time. I took advantage of the special pricing afforded the members of the EMO and joined Lifestyle Family Fitness. My main purpose was for resistance/weight training. I knew I had the cardiovascular exercise covered since I walk, run, and ride my bike. I've been averaging at least 48 miles per week with my bike group and participate in the YFCC Run/Walk Club on Saturday mornings. The weight training has been challenging, but I'm seeing results already. According to the Tanita measurements, I've reduced my body fat and plan to keep going with this program until I get down to where I need to be. I still have a long way to go, but with Dr. Dan's support, I know it will happen one day.

Five years ago, even three years ago, I never would have believed that I'd complete three 5k's, a 10k, a 15k, a half-marathon, and the Disney marathon or that I'd be riding my bike and preparing to ride a 38-mile road race at the end of March; or that I'd have had the confidence to actually climb the Rock Wall on a cruise ship. In my old life, I would have just stood aside and watched others doing it. I actually can't believe how my life has changed, even now. It's even better since I've met some good friends who share the same goals with me. Participating in the Extreme Makeovers has changed my life forever. Because of all I've learned about proper nutrition, I'll never view food the same way again. I try to educate others around me as I see them put seven sugars in the coffee or eating Mickey-D's for breakfast each morning. They don't listen, but it doesn't stop me from trying to share all I've learned whenever an opportunity arises. And sometimes, they do listen.

Label reading, proper supplementation, and using green cleaning/personal care products will always be a part of my life. Maybe ignorance was bliss because I can never go back to the way I was. This is my journey from here on out. After 52 years, I'm finally happy with my life and plan on being around for another 50 years, utilizing all I've learned at Extreme Makeovers and getting my all-important life-saving adjustments. Thanks for changing my life forever. No limits!

Carol Copeland

Dear Doctor Dan,

I was brought by my wife Nancy to a community dinner. To be honest with you, I really didn't want to come. I fought with her every step of the way. I was mad when I got there and told her there was no way I could be helped. I had tried everything, and all they did was hurt me even more, so I thought this was also a waste if my time and hers. As I sat through the meeting and I saw how Dr. Dan was so passionate and his heart was into what he was saying, I figured I would give him a chance. I was not sure I could be helped and I was tired of being hurt and didn't want to go through it all over again. I thought I was going to live with the pain the rest of my life. But I was wrong, and my new life was just beginning.

The reason I participated was because of Nancy, and I guess there was hope that some of my pain would be relieved. I just wanted to feel better and be able to live life without pain and be able to do what I wanted to do without hurting. I wanted my life back.

As far as achieving my goal, I have gone further than I ever expected. I cannot believe the changes in my body, my mind, my heart, and my soul. I have surpassed every goal I set for myself. I have lost weight, my headraces are gone, my eyesight is much better, and I can walk without pain in my legs, back and neck. I feel like I'm twenty-nine again. I can run again without being out of breath due to my old weight. My joints feel so much better. I have a new outlook on life, thanks to Dr. Dan.

Dr. Dan and staff, I could never begin to thank you for all your support and help. Dr. Dan, you have totally changed my life – and all for the better. I am not a miserable person anymore because of my pain. You have taken it from me, and I will never be able to thank you or show you enough how I feel about you. Thank you for sharing all of your knowledge with us, and I hope to learn more.

Before meeting Dr. Dan, I was injured on a job. There was a toolbox dropped on my head and it weighed 75 pounds. It decompressed my *spine and ruptured four disks in my neck and two in my upper back and two in my lower. It was very painful, and I was on meds for four months but didn't like how they made me feel. I could hardly pick up anything over eight pounds. The M.D. told me I would need my neck operated on, and I refused. Then they said I would have to live with it for the rest of my life. They were totally wrong, thanks to Dr. Dan.*

Dr. Dan, you have changed my life and have given me new hope and a better way of life and I could never repay you for what you have done. You are a very caring man to give so much of your time to help others. God has given you a special talent. You have added so much joy and love into our life. It will remain with us the rest of our lives and close to our hearts.

God bless,

Edward T. Allen

My journey to health:

It's always been a passion of mine. When I was in my twenties, I spent a lot of time in a nursing home with my dad and at that time decided I never wanted to end up like that. So my quest for health has always been of great importance to me.

I must say it has never been quite as intense as now through the Extreme Makeover. I am so amazed to continually learn more and more. Just when I thought I knew it all. I am being forced to go another couple of levels higher to greater health with just enough support to motivate me further. As I think back, this is something I've only dreamed of having. To have the knowledge of Dr. Dan and the support of the whole team, I am in awe. I am so thankful. This is not to say this has been quite the challenge. Unless your back is against the wall, you really don't step up to the plate. My journey here has been quite difficult at times – times when I really wanted some chocolate and sugar, times while going through the detox and wanting to break. I just stay focused on the results. I know there is a pot of gold at the end of the rainbow.

As hard as I have tried on my own for good health, without the knowledge I could not have achieved it alone. I didn't realize the need for cleansing at a cellular level. I have worked with chemicals all my life, and I so much enjoy the activities in my life and plan to continue them all until I'm way into my nineties. So, in my opinion, there is no other choice but to work hard through it all, because I win the prize in the end. The prize is good health. You can have all the money in the world, and if you don't have your health, you don't have anything. Good health enables you to do the things you've dreamed of doing. It gives you a quality of life that is incomparable to anything else. It allows you freedom, which can speak volumes; freedom to be the helper, rather than the one being helped; freedom not only physically, but mentally and emotionally, too. Good health to me is the way God intended it to be. It sets an example for others. It encourages others, and gives hope to them. It's stepping out and being different from others. I've always said yes, I am over the top with my health and nutritious way, but I win in the end.

I am truly thankful for our very giving Dr. Dan. He is definitely over the top, too. It's good to know there are others wanting and desiring the same goal. Thank you, Dr. Dan, and thank you, staff. You all work together as a great team.

Janet B.

I participated in this EMO just for fun with the YFCC screening team. This was my second EMO. My first EMO was a total lifestyle change. Before any EMO, I had changed to organic foods. I also had started to exercise again with water fitness exercises and swimming. But mainly I had started receiving chiropractic care from Dr. Dan and doing my spinal exercises. My first EMO brought me knowledge and tools to achieve more with less effort, but most importantly without injury or damage. I learned a few basics that were missing from my nutrition plan and my fitness challenge. I discovered all the toxins, how to minimize their intake and maximize the cleansing process. I started eating the Green Vibrance and Mila. I integrated the coconut oil and avocados into my meals. I reduced the meat, grains and fruits. Drinking more water with a pinch of sea salt hydrated me, finally! I received three colonics, which liberated my body of the past and allowed me to absorb better. I also made peace with others and myself and adopted a better attitude. All my symptoms faded or disappeared. I now have pain-free menses and clear skin. My body does not ache anymore. I have a better posture, stronger muscles, and way more energy as I sleep better. I can now accomplish five times more in a day and in a week. I can think clearly. I quit coffee the first day of my first EMO. My body is now alkaline. I can now exercise at a constant pace for an hour. I can burst many times in a row for three complete sets of three. As a child, I could not sprint, I could not jog, and I could barely walk without twisting an ankle. The only sport I could do was swimming, and I was always last at the finish line. As an adult, I was involved in three car accidents, three years in a row. I didn't have symptoms right away, but 15 years later I had lower back pain with three herniated disks (MRI was done but nothing suggested to improve); restless leg syndrome; and many other symptoms, like sinus infections, bladder infections, constipation, fatigue, and of course depression. Luckily, I have always been against pills, so I was not taking any. So for my second EMO, it has not been extreme at all. I have just been consistent in my new lifestyle. I joined the Lifestyle Fitness center. I am receiving help from a personal trainer who specializes in rehabilitation. My 12-year-old son and I both have the same posture, so we are going through a program together, doing interval circuits to improve our posture in continuation with Dr. Dan's adjustments and spinal exercises. I am closer to the Arc of Life now. Ten months ago, I had a −1 degree curve in my neck; last month, it was up to +19 degrees, so I am on my way to +43 degrees. My thermal scans used to be unbalanced with a lot of pressure everywhere (multicolor), but I now have an all-white and balanced scan. For my second EMO — now that it is easy for me — I had my children participate more. They are now asking questions about the food before eating it. They exercise more consistently as well. Our daily nutrition includes PaleoBars, Intramax, omegas in balances and fiber (Mila or Vega) with Greens regularly. My weekly exercise include the Run/Walk Club; once-a-week corrective exercise at Lifestyle; twice/week exercise with burst training integrated, mostly jogging on a treadmill or sidewalk. I've also been taking short walks once or twice daily with my dog for the past two years. I take some fresh air, look at nature in the morning, and contemplate the sky at night. I work in my yard and connect with nature. I am no longer a prisoner of my body. I am my greatest asset. I will continue with my new lifestyle to lead the way for others. I am grateful for the Maximized Living Centers and Dr. Dan. Thank you for searching for me and rescuing me. I am blessed to have found you. It is a privilege to be one of Dr. Dan's patients. Now, I also have the honor to be part of his team and serve the community. I experience the difference: No limits!!!

Melanie Martel

How it started: I have a friend (Doris) at work who had some back problems and started going to Dr. Yachter. Doris was starting to look better. She was feeling better, and she always had a water bottle with green stuff in it. All Doris could talk about was this great man (Dr. Dan) and this Extreme Makeover Class that her family was going to. On Tuesdays, Doris would talk about what she learned at the class — great stuff. I was hooked. I knew this man could help Eddie and me. Doris invited Eddie and me to one of Dr. Dan's "Community Dinner with the Doc." It was some night, and we have been blessed to have met this doctor who has taught us how to take care of our bodies, back, hearts, souls, and our temples.

Why we started: It's time for a new life. I was on thyroid and blood pressure meds; thyroid meds for about 1.5 years. My medical doctor said my thyroid was sleeping and we would have to get the numbers up. He said I would be on the medications for the rest of my life. It was the same for my blood pressure meds. I was on three kinds: an antibetablocker, water pill, and something else. I told that doctor that I didn't want to be on the antibetablocker anymore and to get me off of it, but she was not happy. So we tried it, and my blood work was fine. I hate taking pills. I also have problems with my neck. Dr. Dan took pictures of my neck, and yes there are problems — my neck is going the wrong way!

My goals: My goals were to get off all meds. Done! To lose weight: Done! Also, to learn how to take care of myself and Eddie in order to live a happier, healthier, fuller life…Dr. Dan has changed my life. Just a few big things he has taught me. Stop the poisoning such as table salt, white flour and sugar. Cleanse and detoxify; fruits, vegetables and whole grains. Eat mostly foods of plant origin. Revitalize and regenerate by eating food the way God created them, in a natural state not altered by man.

I learned about vitamins, how to read food labels, and to get at least 30 minutes of activity daily (add the burst!). I thank God for you, Dr. Dan and staff, for doing the right thing and getting the knowledge out to us. I am a doer! No limits!

Thanks and God bless,

Nancy Booz

If someone had told me that at age 48, I would be exercising daily, riding hundreds of miles for the past three years on a bike, getting up at 5 a.m. on Saturdays for the Run/Walk Club, doing 5ks, and now a 10k, I would have told that person that they were crazy. But this is my life and I love it. Both Dennis and I have met a lot of friends through Dr. Dan and Run/Walk Club he started just over three years ago. After the club, Dennis had the idea of riding a bike for a few miles which now has turned into 16 miles on Saturdays, 32 miles on Sundays, and we have been getting out a couple of evenings each week to ride, too.

My personal goal was to ride my bike a total of 500 miles from Jan. 1, 2009, through the end of December. After my ride today with Carol Copeland, I now have 385.6 miles on my bike. Some days are hard to get out on the trail, but once we get moving, I feel so much better. Dr. Dan was so right when he said that once you get out there and start moving your body, you would feel great. I love those little endorphins!

Dr. Dan has totally changed my life. Not only is Dr. Dan my chiropractor, but he is my great friend, coach, mentor, and has helped me out over the past few years by teaching me better health through awesome Extreme Makeovers and workshops. I can't tell you how much I have learned over the past few years from each EMO I have attended. I always learn new information from each one.

During this EMO I have learned that I can take time out for just me. I have picked up books and started reading again. It had been years since I actually bought books and took time out for myself to sit down and read, other than doing my Bible study reading.

Dennis and I have not missed a day on our Wii Fit since we bought it 38 weeks ago. I am not up to doing 30 jackknives each day and push-up side planks along with other fitness exercising. We work out every morning and also lift weights and walk daily. It is totally amazing how much energy I have every day. None of this would have been possible without being motivated by Dr. Dan just over three years ago.

I have dropped weight and kept it off for three years now. I have toned up my body; something I never thought would happen. I really like my body and the way I am looking now. I still have a ways to go to look as toned as Jillian Michaels, but I am on a journey and if I never get my body like hers, I will be content to look like I do now.

Thank you, Dr. Dan, for not only teaching and sharing with us at the EMO and the Run/Walk Club, but also taking time out on Mondays for the EMO phone calls. Dennis and I have enjoyed listening to each one. We thank God every day that He brought us to you at the seminar you did at Stetson Baptist Church almost four years ago.

God bless and no limits,

Vicki & Dennis Bruno

IT'S YOUR LIFE. MAKE A CHANGE!

- Eliminate the poisons and toxins in your body that create high blood pressure, heart disease, high cholesterol, high blood sugar, diabetes, inflammation, digestive issues, and immune system dysfunctions.

- Release the stress in your life.

- Watch the fat melt off.

- Learn about the recent Harvard Study that reveals secrets to preventing cancer.

- Learn the essentials for healthy longevity; become the one-in-1,000 person who is healthy, pain-free, and living the life we were meant to live after sixty.

Nutrition: Learn cutting-edge nutritional secrets to personalize your diet based on your specific hormones and cellular function. Learn how to get three times more energy.

HOPE GIVEN, HOPE RECEIVED

Congratulations to all participants of the winter 2009 Extreme Makeover forty-day challenge. The team at YFCC is so proud of you! Your commitment to God, your family, and your health is impressive. No more than 5 percent of the population will ever commit to anything long-term. You have now officially become part of the 5 percent.

The transformations have been absolutely mind-blowing! This EMO has seen more lives changed and saved more than any other.

Some of the spectacular results are as follows:

350 participants

Total (group) weight lost: 372 total pounds lost

Total decrease in Body Mass Index: 29.9

Total decrease in Fat Mass: 195 pounds

Average total increase in Muscle Mass: 29 pounds

Lives radically changed: 350

Medications eliminated: blood pressure medications, caffeine (coffee!), Welbutrin, Nexium, Zocor, muscle relaxers, ibuprofen, Percoset, Lisinopril, hydrochorothiazide, Extra Strength Tylenol, beta-blockers, and Lipitor.

Conditions eliminated (reported by participants): Subluxation, nerve impingement, numbing, burning, tingling, sleep apnea, acid reflux, migraine headaches, varicose veins, dry eye syndrome, obesity, osteoporosis, fatigue, acne, reflux, high blood pressure, high triglycerides, neck and back pain, binge eating, anorexia, bulimia, endometriosis, asthma, allergies, sinus problems, anemia, restless leg syndrome, arthritis, sciatica, swollen glands in neck and arm, memory loss, nausea, foggy thinking, neurotoxicity, anxiety, metal and mold toxicity, hair thinning and hair loss, nail fungus, thyroid disease, runny nose, marital problems, moodiness, irritability, tendonitis, poor eyesight, hot flashes, indigestion, depression, shoulder pain, diabetes, high LDL, low HDL, and dizziness, not to mention that a surgical candidate set to go under a knife for a neck problem was able to cancel his surgery.

Neurotoxic patients: Over fifty participants enrolled in our neuro-detoxification and customized nutrition program. They are now having heavy metals, environmental toxins, biotoxins, and molds cleansed from their bodies. Perhaps it goes without saying, but these issues went undiscovered by all other doctors and offices.

Nerve system exams: Over fifty new patient spinal/nerve system evaluations were performed. These people are now having their subluxations and nerve interference removed so they can express their full human potential.

CHAPTER 10

A BALANCED PERSPECTIVE

The following interviews are from medical doctors that I have the personal privilege of working with. Their views are expressed in the form of interviews and brief statements. One interview is from Gwen Olsen, not a medical doctor, but a former drug representative.

Mike is a medical doctor in Private Anesthesiology Practice since 1995 in Orlando. The following is an interview I had with him recently.

1. In general, what have you seen in medical practice?

In general, anesthesiology (with the exception of the pain management subspecialty) does not involve long-term care of patients. We see patients in an acute care setting, which has both good and bad points. Among the good points is that we immediately see the results of surgical procedures. For instance, when people come to the operating room with bone fractures or significant lacerations involving nerve, ligament or skin and awaken to the feeling of having these insults fixed, it is a feeling of immediate satisfaction for us in the medical/surgical fields. Among the less desirable parts of my field is that, although we can see immediate results, we lose follow-up and do not see the long-term results of our earlier efforts. One theme that is prevalent throughout modern medicine is that people/patients, in general, want immediate results (if not sooner!) that do not require any effort on their part.

2. From your perspective, what is the overarching sentiment in medicine today?

There are several sentiments that dominate medicine today. At the forefront is the fear of a malpractice lawsuit. As a member of the medical field, I realize that genuine malpractice does occur. However, I believe that a doctor is much more likely to be sued over a "bad outcome" rather than malpractice. An example would be the female who is seven months pregnant, inhales a few "hits" of crack cocaine (which can and frequently causes dangerously high blood pressures), and due to these high blood pressures has her placenta separate from the inside of her uterus (a placental abruption). As you can imagine, this can lead to a significant reduction in blood flow to the fetus. (I am using the term "fetus" to describe this baby because, by convention, the term "infant" is reserved for after birth.) This female makes it to the emergency room bleeding from her vagina in time to have an emergency C-section and deliver a brain-damaged infant. Our fear is that a jury will feel sympathy for this new mother and the massive lifelong costs which are required to treat her new baby and, even though there was no medical malpractice that occurred, will award her big bucks from a sympathy standpoint from that "rich doctor."

Another sentiment is the constant battle with the government over proper documentation, the massive amount of paperwork that the government requires and trying to stay in "compliance" with all of these mandates. For example: A man goes into his primary physician's office for a checkup and he and his doctor discover that the man has contracted AIDS or herpes or some other sexually transmitted disease from an affair he is having. The patient informs the doctor that he intends to continue having sexual relations with his wife and he does not want her informed of these test results, even though she is also a patient of the same physician. Because of HIPAA, the physician can face loss of license, a fine (I believe $250,000, but I'm not sure) and prison time for informing the wife of this potentially life-saving information. Actual case: Because of HIPAA, a sixteen-year-old boy refused to allow the doctor to reveal the results of a drug screen the boy had taken after the father drove the boy to the doctor's office for the expressed intent of having him tested for illegal drugs. Sometimes the punishment for doing what is "right" is so steep that one cannot afford to do what is "right."

Next is reimbursement from insurance companies. These companies are always trying to deny payment for care that has already been rendered. They employ tactics such as sending the physician a check for 20 percent of the contracted fee for a procedure with fine print on the check stating that "cashing this check recognizes that this is full payment for services rendered." If the secretary in the office does not catch this, the insurance company saved 80 percent at the expense of the doctor. Another tactic is for the insurance company to inform the patient that their treatment was not covered by their policy. Five to ten percent of people will not fight this, and the insurance company just increased their profits some more. Yet another tactic is to delay payment. If you're a big insurance company and pay out $40 million per month in claims and can delay paying those claims for 120 days – that's a fair amount of interest. Yet another example is, in surgery, if several procedures are performed during the same operation (for example an abdominal aortic aneurysm repair which takes about four hours and pays the surgeon $1,000 and a hernia repair on the same patient which takes about twenty minutes and pays the surgeon about $100), the surgeon will get 100 percent of the primary procedure and 50 percent reimbursement for the secondary procedure. In the aneurysm/hernia surgery the surgeon should get paid $1,050 (100% of $1,000 and 50% of the $100 hernia). The insurance company will call the hernia the primary procedure and the aneurysm the secondary procedure and hope the physician's billing office does not catch the switch. In this case the insurance company pays $600 (100% of the $100 hernia and 50% of the $1,000 aneurysm).

And, of course, there is the problem of reimbursement in general. Most, if not all insurance contracts for physicians' reimbursements are based on Medicare. Medicare is cutting physician reimbursement drastically. For example, a cardiac surgeon told me his Medicare reimbursement for cardiac surgery is down 85 percent from what he got paid fifteen years ago. He now only collects 15 percent of what he collected for the same operation in 1984 – and his expenses have not decreased at all.

3. What is 'right' and what is 'wrong' with medicine today?

Right: Advances in scanning technology (new MRI technology, etc), advances in clinical trials and research, advances in new surgical techniques (computer assisted total joint replacements, real time MRI guided sinus and neurosurgery)

Wrong: Frivolous medical malpractice suits, the costs of the new technologies, the influence insurance companies have over patient decision-making (pressure to not refer patients to specialists), questionable practices from drug companies with the FDA in getting drugs approved. (Of note: I understand the need for the high costs of these new drugs and pieces of equipment. A patent will last for, I believe,

17 years. By the time a drug company has spent twelve years and $700,000,000 (yes, seven hundred million) to get a drug approved, the company must make up all the research money for that drug, plus all the money spent on drugs that did not meet FDA approval, in the five years left before the patent expires.) Another big problem with medicine is the fact that we are now an impatient society. We want results now (if not sooner), and it's better if these results do not require any effort on our parts. Physicians will lose patients if they do not prescribe a pill for the patients' conditions (even with the full knowledge that the pill will provide no benefit other than psychological (which is pretty powerful itself). HIPAA & JCAHO also suck! Although their original intention was noble, they have been so "bastardized" by governmental regulation that the initial intents are almost totally obscured.

4. What is the proper way one should 'utilize' the medical profession?

Obviously, trauma should be treated immediately.

The best way to utilize modern medicine is with prevention. I recommend these "lifescans." They can diagnose a variety of potentially very bad conditions and can catch them early. For example, we had a patient come in for an elective repair of an abdominal aortic aneurysm repair when one was diagnosed on one of these scans. That patient's father had died of a ruptured abdominal aortic aneurysm. Many of these conditions are caused by "screw-ups" in the genetic blueprint used to create the proteins that are the building blocks of the body. For example: It is a multistep process to make the myelin sheaths that surround nerves. The raw building blocks of this final product go through many enzymatic processes to reach the final product. If there is an error in the formation of any of these intermediary substrates (i.e. an error in the genetic code that creates the enzyme to take one substrate to the next) then the final product may or may not be compatible with life.

In summary, prevention is the best way medicine should be utilized. If prevention is not used or a condition cannot be avoided even with early diagnosis, then treatment is the next step.

5. Where do you see health-care heading in the near and far future?

Unfortunately, because of the increased costs of the new technologies and the fact that there are so many lawyers in Washington, D.C., I feel that we will have both rationing of health care and little chance of tort reform. Because of the threat of medical malpractice suits, many tests are ordered to try to find that 1 in 1,000,000 diagnosis. Because if that patient, who shows up with the same symptoms that the prior 100 patients had (all of whom had "strep throat"), actually has acute myelogenous leukemia, and you miss it – you just bought someone a house!

6. What do you do to keep your family healthy?

We eat well, exercise moderately, load up on antioxidants, practice prevention and homeopathy, and, of course, adhere to a regular course of weekly chiropractic adjustments.

7. What would you recommend to other families in terms of achieving and maintaining health and vitality?

The same. It's really not complicated. It is a lifestyle choice of health and prevention.

NAME: JOSEPH A CANNIZZARO, M.D., NMD

University of Bologna (1970-1977); School of Medicine & Surgery; Bologna, Italy; MD Cum Laude

MEDICAL STAFF PRIVILEGES: Florida Hospital Medical Center: Orlando, Winter Park, Altamonte Springs, Active medical staff 1981-present

Dr. Cannizzaro shares his thoughts on health care:

Medicine is in need of healing. We are experiencing soul loss in medicine; a lack of a sense of belonging to a community of commitment and shared intent which is at the core of the integrity of the profession. Holistic, integrative, natural medicine can return medicine to its innate wholeness and power, its direction, meaning, and purpose, and integrate the potential for healing with the expertise and technology of curing. Integration of doctor-patient roles into healing teams is the true essence of holistic, natural medicine. Awareness, acceptance, and sharing of conscious and unconscious belief systems and therapies in open dialogue in a nontraditional way are key factors to accomplish this integration. Patients become active partners responsible for their health and become empowered to maintain their health.

Dr. Yachter and I encourage the investigation, recognition, and acceptance of the spiritual component in the healing process and the value of both reasoning and intuition in medical care. The 'new medicine' allows us to modify gene expression with the new therapeutic tools: nutrition, exercise, mind-body medicine, nutraceuticals, chiropractic care, and traditional healing systems. All education programs and offerings are designed to incorporate the timeless wisdom of nature and the ancient healing traditions, modern science, and transformative practice. With this integration of theory and embodied practice, our students and community members learn to cultivate a healing presence and create optimal healing environments in all areas of their lives

Dr. Dan Yachter wholeheartedly exemplifies these principles in his practice and I've had the privilege of integratively collaborating with him in caring of our mutual patients. We've gone a long way together to bring about optimal health and well-being with this model.

OUR FAVORITE PEDIATRICIAN

"Dr. Cannizzaro is one of the best pediatricians, as he is not a fan of stuffing pills and antibiotics into our children to cover up symptoms. His advice and genuine regard for our son has been helpful and appreciated. He has helped us deal with ailments and encouraged us to live healthy – promoting good health first. My son's sensitivities to drugs has been an issue, and I always know that Dr. C will attend to his needs and health in a manner that makes us regard him as family! ---one of Dr. Cannizzaro's patients

From Gwen Olsen:

She spent 15 years as a sales rep in the pharmaceutical industry working for health-care giants such as Johnson and Johnson and Bristol-Myers Squibb. Gwen is currently a writer, speaker, and natural health consultant.

THE UNHOLY MARRIAGE TO
AMERICAN HEALTH CARE

It appears people have married the health-care system in this country. Americans are either unconvinced or unwilling to acknowledge that our health-care system is corrupt, underserving, unmanageable and outright dangerous. (By way of example, we are reducing our cholesterol with statin drugs and bombarding our immune systems with live viruses, debris, and other neurotoxins annually to prevent influenza.) In other words, the majority of us have taken some sort of sacred oath to continue to adhere to the ludicrous practices we currently call health care "for better or for worse...until death do us part." As a consequence, a large number of us are fulfilling those vows. A very large number of us are dying at the hands of our own health-care system!

When I left the pharmaceutical industry in 2000 to enter the natural foods industry, I never dreamed that many of the health symptoms I suffered from were directly related to my access to and use of the health-care system I had worked in for fifteen years. Since then, I have discovered nearly all of my major health challenges and related problems over the years were the result of my own ignorance, false programming, and indoctrination by a "sick care" health model. Mainly, however, it was my own indiscriminate and unnecessary use of prescription drugs – my "quick fix, pop-a-pill" mentality – that had almost killed me on more than one occasion.

The United States recently ranked a disgustingly low nineteenth in preventable deaths among industrialized nations. However, our health-care spending is 16 percent of our gross domestic product, causing grave concern for third-party payers and government-backed health programs such as Medicare and Medicaid. Taxpayers spent over $2.1 trillion on health care in 2006 with a large portion of that attributable to Medicare drug benefits. Baby boomers are aging rapidly, and price increases for health-care services and drugs far outpace cost-of-living wage increases, so many Americans are already feeling the financial crunch associated with costly health care. Not to mention, there are a projected 45 million Americans who are completely without health insurance coverage.

New information surfaces daily where drug manufacturers have covered up damning evidence about their blockbuster drugs – having waited years (sometimes decades) before disclosing information in the discovery process of lawsuits about side effects that were evident early on in their initial clinical trials. Yet, we continue to allow new drugs to be advertised in direct-to-consumer ads on TV and in every other form of media, while only one other country on the planet permits direct advertising influence on consumers by drug companies—New Zealand.

There's a very good reason for that: Direct-to-consumer ads drive branded product market share because patients ask for specific drugs by name. However, drugs are not benign products such as Band Aids or Kleenex. All drugs are toxins and have the potential to harm, maim, and/or kill people. Even drugs considered benign such as aspirin and Tylenol can be deadly. Doctors should be the sole recipients of any advertising provided by drug manufacturers, and even their exposure should be limited to true, fair, and balanced medical information about the products rather than the Madison Avenue marketing spin.

So, where is our voice – the voice of we the people? Why are we tolerating this deception and corruption while the body counts climb higher and higher and the corporations get richer and richer? Why aren't we screaming at the tops of our lungs? Have we all lost our minds and simply refuse to accept responsibility for something we have created that is not working, an archaic institution whose conflicts of interest have become detrimental to our well-being as individuals and to our society as a whole?

I say let's admit our failure and move on. Let's sever the ties with the old and find a better fit for the future. We need a system geared toward prevention and wellness rather than symptom management and disease maintenance. We need a system based on accountability and sound judgment that nurtures competition. We need regulators who are not financially influenced by the industries they are tasked to regulate. And the American people need to take their calcium and grow a backbone and push back against these atrocities with their legislators!

The pharmaceutical industry has roughly 1,100 lobbyists to represent their interests in Washington. Do you know how many congressmen and senators we, the people, have representing us? Less than half that number. Do you know who your representatives are and with whom to voice your opinion and make it count? If not, whose voice do you think is resounding in the corridors and ears of your legislators: the people's voice, or Pharma's paid mouthpieces?

When divorce in the United States is said to be about 50 percent of couples, I find it hard to believe that we are so doggedly committed to our values and belief systems that we would stay in a relationship that is abusive and even deadly out of convenience. But we do it every day in this country by refusing to take part in health care and political reform, and by standing by idly while our loved ones and the world we once knew disintegrate in the hands of an incompetent and corrupt few. We are the masses. The numbers are on our side.

An infamous mass murderer in history knew the paralyzing effect that large numbers of dead and dying people have on the masses. Joseph Stalin was quoted as having said, "One death is a tragedy. A thousand deaths is a statistic." My fear is that Americans have become numb to the large-scale tragedy, depicted in the numbers of dead and dying, that we now refer to as health care.

DRUGGING OUR CHILDREN TO DEATH:
BY GWEN OLSEN

In Massachusetts, a four-year-old girl named Rebecca became the center of a murder investigation after being found dead from an overdose of a dangerous combination of drugs. Her parents and psychiatrist are facing criminal prosecution and will stand trial later this year.

In Florida, a seven-year-old boy named Gabriel made headlines because he hanged himself with a shower hose in his foster home. It was later discovered that the boy was on an unauthorized cocktail of psychiatric drugs while in the state's protective custody. He had been taken from his mother, who was herself deemed a danger to the child because of drug addiction.

In Texas, a fourteen-year-old boy named Matthew died suddenly after only 29 days on a powerful stimulant for ADHD. His devastated parents are suing the drug manufacturer and were recently interviewed on ABC's Good Morning America.

The New York Times profiled a prominent Harvard psychiatrist, Joseph Biederman, whose claim to fame was the popularization of bipolar disorder in adolescents and children. Biederman's research contributed to a fortyfold increase in the diagnoses of pediatric bipolar disorder from 1994 to 2003. However, he is accused of failing to report nearly $1.6 million in pharmaceutical manufacturers' consulting fees he collected from the years 2000 to 2007, according to information given to congressional investigators. His "oversight" was uncovered by U.S. Sen. Charles Grassley's investigative committee.

The National Institutes of Health and the Food and Drug Administration released a study featured in the American Journal of Psychiatry that found children and teens who died suddenly were 7.4 times more likely than not to have been taking stimulant medications.

These are all taken from recent headlines. These are national current events.

The onslaught of direct-to-consumer advertising to parents and educators about the benefits of stimulant drugs designed for focusing attention and curbing misbehavior has resulted in a large number of deaths and injuries to our nation's children. And to what benefit? Even the most recent follow-up results of the prestigious Multimodal Treatment Study of Children with ADHD, funded by the National Institute of Mental Health, concluded that any minor benefits exhibited by stimulant drug use in the initial treatment stages of ADHD symptoms in children were not sustained in the long term.

The black-boxed warnings added to stimulant treatments for ADHD, antidepressants, atypical anti-psychotics, mood stabilizers and anti-seizure drugs all indicate a causal link between these drugs and suicide. Some package inserts even contain warnings related to violence and homicide. Most labels warn of the possibility of experiencing anxiety, sleeplessness, aggression, loss of appetite, agitation, depression, hallucinations and psychosis.

Nearly all psychiatric drugs have withdrawal and addiction potential, as well as links to other serious illnesses including endocrine issues like excessive weight gain and diabetes. Yet, these drugs are marketed and prescribed nonchalantly to our children – even our toddlers – to control behavior. Is it because the drugs' benefits truly exceed their risks (in what is known as the risk-to-benefit ratio evaluation of treatment)? Or, is it really because our children have been identified as the most lucrative expansion market available to the pharmaceutical industry?

Children are known to be compliant patients and that makes them a highly desirable market for drugs, especially when it pertains to large-profit-margin psychiatric drugs, which can be wrought with issues of noncompliance because of their horrendous side-effect profiles but require no medical tests to diagnose the disorders for which these drugs are prescribed.

Children are forced by school personnel to take their drugs, they are forced by their parents to take their drugs, and they are forced by their doctors to take their drugs. So, children are the ideal patient type because they represent refilled prescription compliance and "longevity." In other words, they will be lifelong patients and repeat customers for Pharma.

Branded drugs representing $17 billion in sales lost their exclusivity in 2007. Even though sales grew 3.8 percent and totaled $286.5 billion, "the U.S. pharmaceutical market experienced its lowest growth rate since 1961," said IMS Health's Murray Aitken, senior vice president of health-care insight. Manufacturers are scrambling to make up these lost revenues just as the average American further tightens his belt in anticipation of a downward spiraling economy.

As insured patient populations capable of paying for exorbitantly priced pharmaceuticals diminish, the importance of government mandated vaccinations, government funded health programs such as Medicare and Medicaid, and mandatory mental health screenings that result in prescription psychotropic drug sales will all increase in value to Pharma. Sales managers must search for ways to expand market share. As a consequence, Pharma's lobbyists will intensify their efforts in capitals across America to promote government-endorsed programs funded by taxpayers that have a guaranteed reimbursement plan¬¬ – no matter what price the manufacturers choose to charge.

In fact, more money was spent on the treatment of mental disorders for children ages 17 and under than was spent on any other medical condition in 2006. That year, as reported by the Agency for Healthcare Research and Quality on April 22, 2009, total expenses for mental health treatment totaled $8.9 billion.

In the April issue of Pediatrics, the government's U.S. Preventive Services Task Force urged physicians to routinely screen all American teens for depression. However, the unscientific questionnaires produce a high rate of false mental illness diagnoses. Diagnosis equals treatment recommendation. Treatment equals drugs and exposes our children to the dangers of mind-altering chemicals that have been proved to have only nominal efficacy.

The initiative to drug our children for profit has exceeded all common-sense boundaries and is threatening the welfare of every American child. It is up to each and every one of us to stop this madness. We have allowed ourselves to be sold down the river by savvy marketing executives who care more about their corporate bottom line than they do about our children or our families. The scope of the collective greed and malice has now reached epidemic proportions and, sadly enough, can be measured in body counts – many of them being our children's.

The numbers don't lie. The verdict is in. We are drugging our children to death!

APPENDIX

YFCC Clinical Resources

- Health workshops such as: nutrition, fitness, water, time and stress management are offered as well as customized nutrition, detoxification, and how to raise healthy, drug-free children

- Six-week Extreme Makeovers and one day Makeovers

- Neurotoxicity and Biotoxicity programs to help identify and eliminate deadly toxins from the body

- Patient Appreciation Days (call office for details: 407-333-2277)

- Workshops performed at your business, organization, church, temple, or club.

- Radio program broadcasts on 950 am WTLN: go to our website: yachterhealth.com for program day and time

- Website resources and our TV program available at yachterhealth.com

- Weekly newsletter available for sign-up at yachterhealth.com

- Therapeutic massage care

- YFCC Team Catalyst Run/Walk Club, meeting every Saturday morning at 6:45 a.m. at Panera Bread in Lake Mary and Leesburg

- Nutritional supplements and customized nutrition

- Healthy food products

- Educational books, DVDs, CDs, newsletters, and e-mails

I'm available to come to schools, businesses, civic organizations, churches, temples, and synagogues to speak and teach on any and all principles taught in this book. Extreme Makeover events are available as well for the above-mentioned groups. Please call 407-687-9573 to book an event.

Internet resources

Our practice: **http://www.YACHTERHEALTH.com**

Phenomenal workshop materials, cd's, dvd's:
Health and fitness membership website:

To register, go to: healthandfitnessmembership.com

Gain unlimited access to:

- How-to articles, audios, and videos

- Healthy recipes

- New content, added weekly to expand and inform your healthy world.

Kangen water. Clean water is one of the most important needs of our bodies. For more information, contact:

Toy L. Hightower

United Power Int'l Founder

407-709-3535

www.unitedpowerintl.com

toyhightower@gmail.com

pHmiracleliving.com is a phenomenal resource for alkaline products and lifestyle information. You can also purchase books from Dr. Robert O. Young. His books are powerful documents substantiating the life-transforming benefits of the alkalarian lifestyle.

Vega/Sequel Naturals is a high-quality, plant-based protein/meal replacement supplement. The best I've been able to find. Go to www.yachterhealthsolutions.com to order.

Green Vibrance: Highest quality green food supplement on the market. Contains Superfoods such as chlorella, spirulina, sea vegetables, broccoli sprouts, sunflower sprouts, wheat grass, and various greens powders. Order at: www.yachterhealthsolutions.com

Intramax: Superior Liquid multi-vitamin formula. Go to yacherhealthsolutions.com to order.

Whole Body Vibration.

Vibe Plates: www.yachterhealthsolutions.com

X-iser, a burst training stair-stepper-type apparatus. For amazing burst-type, interval training workouts, check it out at: **www.yachter-healthsolutions.com**

http://gwenolsen.com: Phenomenal resource for the true mission and vision of the pharmaceutical companies in U.S. and beyond. Her book, Confession of an RX Drug Pusher, is an excellent read. It provides excellent information on pharmaceutical medications and their side effects.

High energy quick-tip page:

- Eat every 2-4 hours for maximum energy

- Best not to eat 2-3 hours before bed

- Dairy and gluten destroy energy

- Vitamins B6, B9, B12 boost brain power and decrease brain inflammation

Summary health tips

- Exercise regularly: Some form of burst training and cardio at least three times a week.

- Drink lots of water: It's Mother Nature's most versatile medicine.

- Get six to nine hours of sleep daily.

- Meditate.

- Buy locally grown, organic goods, preferably in season, as often as you can.

- Take nutritional supplements: whole food supplements, organic vitamins, Intramax.

- Use a comprehensive, organically bound, liquid multi-vitamin, and vitamin C.

- Enjoy one hour of full exposure to intense natural sunlight on a near-daily basis with no sunscreen (essential for mental health, bone density, and vitamin D production).

- Try to make your first choice of health-care practitioner an actual practitioner of health care and not sick care.

- Don't follow the USDA's ridiculous Food Guide Pyramid.

- Don't take steroids or other questionable bodybuilding supplements.

- No diet pills, stimulants, or fat-burning pills.

- No fad dieting.

Dr. Dan's list of energy-destroying foods to be avoided

- Sodium nitrite (can cause cancer)

- MSG/monosodium glutamate

- Yeast extract (can cause obesity and nerve damage)

- Hydrogenated oils (can cause heart disease)

- High-fructose corn syrup

- Sugar

- Sucrose (can cause diabetes and obesity)

- Artificial colors (can cause behavioral disorders)

- Aspartame (can cause brain damage, optic nerve damage)

- Homogenized milk fats (can cause heart disease and cardiovascular disorders)

- Commercialized, grain-fed red meat (absolutely no beef, pork, or other red meat)

- Processed cows' milk, cheese, and dairy products

- Soft drinks, junk foods, snack foods, or fast foods

- Processed foods such as cookies, crackers, and frozen dinners

- Fried foods

- White flour and any foods containing white flour

- Refined carbohydrates such as breads, cereals, pastries, and pizza dough

- Fruit juice drinks

- Brand-name laundry detergents (loaded with toxic fragrance chemicals)

- Popular deodorants (contain aluminum)

- Fluoride toothpaste (fluoride is a dangerous ingredient)

- Popular shampoos, soaps, and conditioners (all contain harmful fragrance chemicals)

- Dryer sheets (contain fragrance chemicals)

- Suntan lotions

Dr. Dan's Top Supplement Picks:

- Multivitamins: Intramax

- Superfood supplement: Green Vibrance, Mila, Supergreens

- Hemp and plant-based formula protein shakes: Vega/Sequel Naturals.

- Sea salt: Himalayan Crystal Salt, Celtic Sea Salt, and Real Salt

- Personal care: Organix South and Pangea Organics

- Pet products: OnlyNaturalPet.com

- House cleaning products: Seventh Generation and Dr. Bronner's

Seventh Generation Cleaning and Personal Products

http://www.seventhgeneration.com

Seventh Generation is committed to becoming the world's most trusted brand of authentic, safe, and environmentally responsible products for a healthy home. Seventh Generation brand-name products include: non-chlorine-bleached, 100 percent recycled paper towels, bathroom and facial tissues and napkins; nontoxic, phosphate-free cleaning, dish and laundry products; plastic trash bags made from recycled plastic; chlorine-free baby diapers, training pants, and baby wipes; and chlorine-free feminine care products, including organic cotton tampons. Due to heavy products, best place to buy is at your local whole foods market.

Dr. Dan's recipes for health:

- Fresh green juice feasting

- Quinoa (boiled, used as cereal or soup base)

- Hemp products

- Almond milk

- Healthy oils from raw avocados, extra virgin coconut oil, macadamia nuts, cashews, almonds, flaxseed, and olives

- Massive quantities of vegetables: salad greens, cilantro, broccoli, cabbage, carrots, snow peas, okra, tomatoes, and zucchini.

- Raw, fresh fruits, especially berries (massive quantities of blueberries)

- Healing foods such as garlic, ginger, and onions.

Dr. Dan's daily breakfast or lunch with Green Vibrance shake: (serves up to 2)

Blend all ingredients together in blender:

1 avocado

1 lime (cut in fours – use the "meat")

1 grapefruit (same as lime)

1-2 handfuls of fresh spinach

1 seedless (English) cucumber, peeled

½ can organic coconut milk

1-2 scoops green powder (Green Vibrance or supergeens)

1 scoop Mila/chia seed

1 tablespoon coconut fat/oil

Stevia or agave nectar to sweeten

*optional: peppermint oil/extract

alkalized/ionized/microclustered Kangen water or almond milk to liquefy, if needed ice

Dr. Dan's grocery list

The staples my wife and I buy each week (organic as much as possible) are:

Avocados

Cucumbers

Fresh spinach

Grapefruit

Limes

Apples

Pears

Berries

Broccoli

Cauliflower

Edamame (in and out of pods)

Red/purple cabbage

Lettuce/spring mix

Red onion

Garlic

Tomatoes

Brussels sprouts

Raw nuts (almonds, walnuts, cashews)

Raw seeds (pumpkin, sunflower)

Nut milks (almond, hazelnut)

Hemp milk

Coconut milk

Nut butters

Additionally, my wife and I buy different vegetables (frozen and fresh) each week, depending on availability and season:

Eggplant

Squash

Zucchini

Sweet peas

Turnip greens

Kale

Occasionally I buy:

Amy's Organic soups

(Sprouted) Ezekiel bread (spelt, amaranth, millet)

Raw cheeses

Garbanzo beans (for hummus)

Tuna (for salad)

Cage-free eggs

Organic bison

Udo's Choice Perfected Oil Blend

Go to Yachterhealthsolutions.com to order

Udo's Choice Oil Blend is a carefully blended mix of the finest Omega 3, 6, and 9 varieties of essential fatty acid sources. This premium-quality product has a pleasant light nutty flavor and is easily mixed with health shakes and protein drinks or added as a topping to salads and vegetables. Udo's Choice Perfected Oil Blend is pressed at a temperature of less than 50 degrees Celsius and, more importantly, in the absence of light and oxygen. The use of nitrogen-flushed, amber glass bottles further protects the oil from light and oxygen and helps to ensure maximum stability.

Health Provider Search Tools:

Mercury Free Dentists

http://www.iaomt.org/patients/index.asp

To help you find a mercury-free dentist who will safely remove and replace mercury amalgam (silver) fillings, visit the world's largest database of mercury-free dentists. The database is easy to use and searches for mercury-free dentists by country, state/province, and city. If you live in Orlando area/Seminole County/Lake Mary, I strongly recommend Dr. Nick Brand of Brand New Smiles. His office phone number is 407-862-3344. Address: 1325 S. International Pkwy., Suite 1201, Lake Mary, FL 32746-1406. He is experienced in mercury-free dentistry.

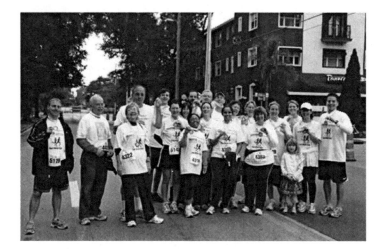

*Picture of the YFCC Team Catalyst Run/Walk Club. (We meet at 6:45 a.m. every Saturday at Panera Bread in Lake Mary.)

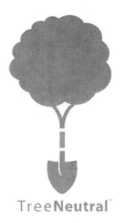

TreeNeutral™